DR SEBI DIET

The Ultimate Alkaline Diet to Help You Lose Weight and Detox Your Body Using 100+ Simple and Quick recipes

Sophia Parks

Table of Contents

Introduction:

Dr. Sebi is a well-known pathologist, naturalist, biochemist and herbalist. He visited different areas from Central and South America, Africa, North America, and the Caribbean. He made a lot of research and personally experienced several herbs; based on his research, he developed a specific approach and deduced technique for curing different diseases affecting the human body by using herbs deeply rooted in more than 30 years of practice.

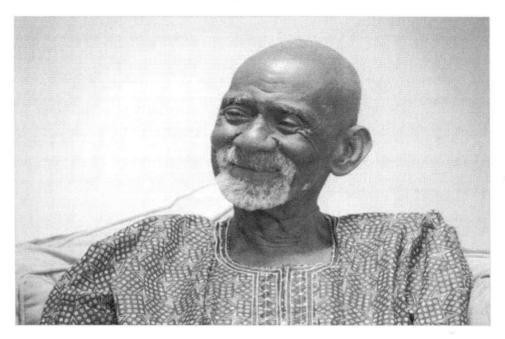

Dr. Sebi is also known as a self-educated person and was diagnosed with asthma, diabetes, obesity and impotence. Sebi firstly came to the United States. He started to become famous as an herbalist in Mexico after his failed treatments with mainstream doctors and their traditional ways of treating medical issues with medicine. From his illnesses and self-experiences with medication based on herbs, he finds noticeable healing progress in his body. This gives birth to an idea for the development of natural food compounds. This food's aim was specifically linked to the body's intercellular cleaning and revitalizing all vital cells responsible for making up the human body. In more than 30 years of Sebi's life, he devoted himself to creating a specific approach that he could acquire through years of scientific experience. He started to share the compounds and his findings with others, which gave birth to a famous Dr. Sebi's Cell Food, motivated by his personal experience and expertise he acquired.

Alkaline foods are considered some of the healthiest foods that exist on earth. These are highly recommended to those suffering from chronic diseases because of the compromised immune system, low energy, anxiety, and headaches. On top of the list red meat, pasta, candies, and dairy products are those foods which cause acid in the body are typically consumed more than other products. It's not an easy task to change someone's diet, especially in those cases when it's supposed to be a sudden or dramatic change. You need to find a solution and ways to agree to someone to change his/her routine to lower the acid load in the body and follow healthy habits regarding eating routines and diet plans to enhance health. There are many dieting debates between the latest diet documentaries and other influencers promoting their current favorite diet pills. With lots of contradictory facts about which food and diet are better, even if it is advocated by somebody who seems credible, it is difficult to differentiate reality from fiction. For example, take Sebi's Diet, which is also 2019's second most-searched diet on Google. Many might assume that this is a physician's created software. It is also assumed that Alfredo Bowman, the founder, was an herbalist, not a medical doctor. Dr. Sebi Diet is highly restrictive in nature, with a lack of protein intake and some vitamins. It mainly focuses on consuming a plant-based diet and avoid refined foods. Dr. Sebi believed that most diseases are caused by mucus and an increased amount of acidity in the body. He argued that by using an alkaline-based food, diseases could not occur.

His plans include a quite stringent dietary routine and costly supplements, which promises to detoxify the human body and prevent it from different diseases and restore alkalinity in the body. Dr. Sebi claims that His Diet plans can greatly help fight against several common diseases, including High blood pressure, diabetes, obesity, liver disorder, kidney problems and many others, which will be discussed in upcoming chapters.

Chapter 1. Dr. Sebi Diet

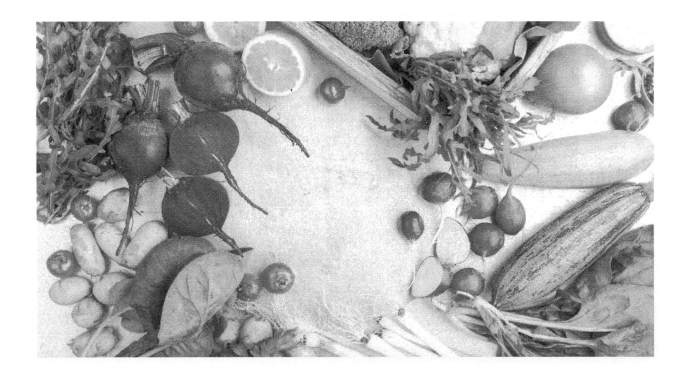

Alkaline foods are considered some of the healthiest foods that exist on earth. These are highly recommended to those suffering from chronic diseases because of a compromised immune system, low energy, anxiety, and headaches. On top of the list red meat, pasta, candies, and dairy products are those foods which cause acid in the body are typically consumed more than other products. It's not an easy task to change someone's diet, especially in those cases when it's supposed to be a sudden or dramatic change. You need to find a solution and ways to agree with someone to change his/her routine to lower the acid load in the body and follow healthy habits regarding eating routines and diet plans to enhance health. There are many dieting debates between the latest diet documentaries and other influencers promoting their current favorite diet pills. With lots of contradictory facts about which food and diet are better, even if it is advocated by somebody who seems credible, it is difficult to differentiate reality from fiction. For example, take Sebi's Diet, which is also 2019 's second most-searched diet on Google. Many might assume that this is a physician's created software. It is also assumed that Alfredo Bowman, the founder, was a herbalist, not a medical doctor. Dr. Sebi Diet is highly restrictive in nature, with a lack of protein intake and some vitamins. It mainly focuses on consuming a plant-based diet and avoid refined foods. Dr. Sebi believed that most diseases are caused by mucus and an increased amount of acidity in the body. He argued that by using an alkaline-based food, diseases could not occur.

1.1 What is the alkaline diet of Doctor Sebi?

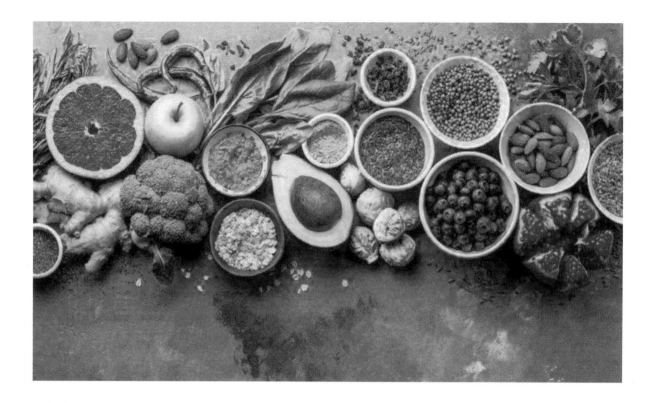

A famous plant-based diet plan has been formulated by late Dr. Sebi, known by his name the Sebi's diet, also known as a Sebi's alkaline diet. This diet helps by removing toxic waste in the body by alkalizing the blood. It is believed that this process revitalizes your cells. The diet normally depends, along with several supplements, on consuming a limited list of approved foods. Dr. Sebi claimed that for more than 400 years, Western medical science is treating sicknesses incorrectly, with very rare cures being noticed. Sebi claimed that diseases are caused by the host being infected due to treatment practices using chemicals because this technique was adopted inherently flawed in society. As a more effective and intuitive approach, Dr. Sebi disproves this technique by referring to African philosophy, normally called African Bio-mineral Balance. The method promoted by Sebi suggests that if a mucous-membrane gets damaged, diseases are induced in the body. A drastic build-up of this mucus is produced when this happens, which in turn creates a disease. So, what is Sebi's answer or what is the alternate way to cope with the problem?

The prevention of these mucus build-ups issue in the body depends on diet. The famous African Bio-mineral Balance philosophy assumes that illness can occur in an acidic climate only. The remedy recommended by Dr. Sebi is to develop a diet plan that mainly focuses on developing an alkaline deficiency. Like many other modern diets, plants are more concentrated with alkaline; because plants are naturally alkaline.

Dr. Sebi asserts that alkaline diet develops an atmosphere in which infection can not flourish. He also argues that African Bio-mineral-Balance rejuvenates damaged body cell tissue. Dr. Sebi has developed a detoxification cleanse process that will purify every cell of the body. the expectation is that, the human body will begin cell rejuvenation process. His alkaline diet, which is mainly based on the famous theory of African Bio-Mineral was developed by Alfredo Darrington Bowman, also self-educated herbalist known best as Dr. Sebi. Although Sebi was not really a medical doctor and he did not hold any doctorate degree. Without depending on standard Western medicine, Sebi built this diet for everyone who wishes to naturally cure or prevent illness and improve health.

As per Dr. Sebi, sickness in an area of the body is the product of mucus build-up. Build-up of mucus, for instance, is pneumonia, whereas diabetes is excess mucus in the pancreas. He claims that in an alkaline setting, diseases do not exist and start to arise when the body is more acidic. He claims to restore the body's normal alkaline condition and detoxify the infected body by closely observing his routine using his expensive supplements. Originally, Dr. Sebi believed that this diet could treat diseases like HIV, sickle cell anemia, leukemias, and lupus. Sebi's diet contains a detailed list of items that have been approved by Sebi. The diet is considered a "vegan diet" the reason is that animal products are not allowed. Dr.Sebi believed that for a human body to heal itself, one must follow the diet faithfully for the remaining of your life. Finally, while many individuals believe that the program has cured them, no scientific findings support these statements. but still the Sebi diet plans are famous all over the world with many positive reviews available on internet.

1.2 How to start and what are the basic principles of this diet:

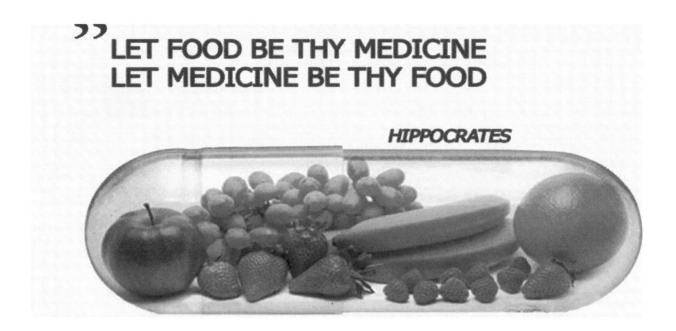

Dr. Sebi believed that diseases are the product of increased mucus and more acidity in body; he claimed that diseases will not occur in alkaline climate. His method, which requires a very restricted diet and effective supplements, promises to purify and restore alkalinity levels in the body (no scientific evidence is able to help his promises).

On the website of Sebi, the guidelines of the diet are quite strict and illustrated in details. You must obey these main guidelines, according to Sebi's dietary guide:

Rule 1. Only the foods specified in the dietary guide must be consumed.

Rule 2. Drink 3.8 liters (1 gallon) of water per day.

Rule 3: Take the supplements an hour before medication.

Rule 4: No animal product allowed.

Rule 5: It does not allow any alcohol.

Rule 6: Stop wheat items and consume only the "natural-growing grains" referred to in the guide.

Rule 7: Don't kill your food. Avoid microwave use.

Rule 8: Stop canned fruits or seedless ones.

There seem to be no clear rules on nutrients. Nevertheless, this diet has low protein, as lentils, beans, and animal products are forbidden. For strong muscles, skin, and body joints, protein is an essential nutrient. Besides, Sebi's listed food products, which are nutrients rich and promise to clean your body and replenish your cells, are still expected to be purchased. The "all-inclusive" kit (search on web), which includes 20 different items that are said to purify and heal your body just at the quickest possible rate, is recommended to be purchased. Besides this, no clear guidelines for supplements are given. Instead, you are supposed to order any medication that suits your health concern. Just for example, "Bio Ferro" capsules tend to treat liver problems, cleanses your bloodstream, improve immunity, encourage weight loss, help digestive problems, and enhance overall well-being. Besides, the supplements do not provide a comprehensive list of ingredients or quantities, making it somehow difficult to understand whether they can do what they are supposed to do. The diet limits animal products while, focuses on vegan food, but with far more strict guidelines. It limits seedless fruits. For instance, it only allows Sebi's approved list of "normal growing grains."

Here is a short description of the foods items that his dietary guide recommends:

Vegetables: use amaranth greens, eat sea vegetables, avocado, garbanzo, bell peppers, beans, chayote, cucumber, izote, kale, lettuce (all but iceberg), onions, nopales, okra, olives, zucchini, squash, tomatoes (only cherry and plum), tomatillo, turnip greens, cress, purslane, wild arugula. Vegetables:

Fruits: apples, bananas, berries (all kinds, not cranberries), elderberries, cantaloupe, dates, figs, currants, grapes, lime, mango peaches, oranges, plums, prickly pears, papayas, peaches, pears, prunes, grapes (seeded), light coconut jelly, soursops, tamarind, etc.

Herbal teas: Burdock, elderberry, chamomile, fennel, ginger, raspberry and tila.

Grains: amaranth, fonio, wheat, spelled, tef, wild rice, Kamut, quinoa.

Nuts and seeds: 'tahini' butter of raw sesame seeds, hemp seeds, raw sesame seeds, walnuts, Brazil nuts.

Oils: olive oil (not cooked), coconut oil (not cooked), grape seed oil, sesame oil, hemp oil, avocado oil.

Seasonings /spices: basil, bay leaf, garlic, dill, oregano, savory, estragon, onion powder, thyme, achiote, cayenne, habanero, pure sea salt, sage, seaweed, pure agave syrup, powder, date sugar.

There is some other rule of the Sebi Food Guide which includes:

Only foods listed in Sebi's Dietary Guide are required to be consumed you have to drink 1 gallon of natural and fresh spring water daily. Alamo's animal products, including fish, dairy, "hybrid" foods, are strictly prohibited. Alcohol is not allowed; the products of the Sebi diet plan must be taken one almost one hour before the pharmaceutical medicines. You have to avoid wheat and consume only the "natural grains" mentioned in the Sebi's Guide. Microwaves must be avoided. Canned foods and seedless fruits are not allowed.

1.3. Advantages and disadvantages of the Doctor Sebi diet

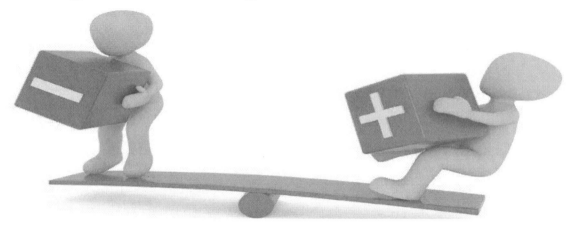

Advantages:

Due to Its heavy focus on a plant-based diet, this is one advantage of the Sebi diet. The diet encourages a huge proportion of fruits and vegetables that are rich in fiber, vitamins, minerals, and plant sources to be eaten.

Significantly lower inflammation & cell proliferation, as well as defenses against many health disorders, have been linked with diets that are rich in fruit content and vegetables. Those who consume seven or even more servings of fruits and veggies each day had a 25% to 31% lower risk of heart-related disease and cancer (based on study of 65,226 individuals).

Moreover, most people do not consume enough dairy food. In a 2017 survey, 9.3 percent and 12.2 percent of individuals met the fruit and veggie guidelines, respectively. Also, the Dr. Sebi diet encourages consuming whole grain food which is rich in fiber and good fats, such as nuts, beans, and vegetable oils. A lower risk of heart disease has been associated with these foods.

Finally, with overall improved diet plan, health can be improved by avoiding and limiting ultra-processed food.

Disadvantages:

This diet is extremely protein deficient: no animal-based products, the eggs, the dairy, even the soy are permitted by Sebi. He limits many other beans and legumes as well. Some hemp seeds, walnuts, natural growing grains, and Brazil nuts are the only things that have some protein in the diet. It can be quite hard to fulfill dietary requirements from these products alone. Protein is a key element of any cell in the human body, and also to help create and heal tissues, the body requires protein. Muscles, skin, blood, and tissue are all an important building block of protein. Nutritional deficiencies and malnourishment can result from constraining major food and nutritional content. While it supports some fruit and veggies, it curiously limits quite a bit of food. It allows for cherry and plum tomatoes, for instance, but no other types. The Iceberg lettuce and the shiitake mushrooms are other types of food that he limits, which makes this diet much more stringent, making it extremely hard to obey.

The primary focus of Sebi is on his products that make big promises that they will "speed up the recovery process" and "rejuvenate and engage intercellular development." Some packages cost well over $1,500 and do not list any nutrient or quantity specifics. This makes it hard to understand what you'll get from his patented blends and also what exactly his supplements contain.

Above all, Dr. Sebi is not a doctor, so there's no evidence-based study to support his statements and directives. his extremely strict dietary recommendations promote the removal of major food groups that can have harmful health effects or, not to forget, can lead to bad relationship to food. It is important to not fall into a dieting conspiracy trap to know the truth and ensure that every diet you adopt is validated by science.

In 1993, after pretending his diet can cure sensitive situations, such as HIV, lupus and leukemia, Dr. Sebi faced litigation. According to Health line, a court asked him to withdraw making such claims. It is crucial to know that there was no PhD obtained by Dr. Sebi. There was also no scientific support for his diet and nutrients. Finally, other unhealthy habits, such as consuming supplements to reach fullness, are promoted by this diet. Since nutrients are not a significant energy source, unhealthy eating habits are guided further by this argument.

Lacks of protein and other key minerals, which are an excellent source of nutrition, are not allowed by Sebi's nutrition guide. Only walnuts, some Brazilian nuts, sesame seeds and hemp seeds that are not rich sources of protein are allowed. For example, 4 grams and 9 grams of protein are given by 1/4 cup (25 grams) of walnuts and 3 tbsp (30 grams) of hemp seeds, accordingly.

You will need to eat incredibly large quantities of such foods to satisfy your protein intake needs. While certain foods, including potassium, beta carotene, and vitamin-C and Vitamin-E, appear high in foods in diet, they are relatively low in omega3, iron, calcium, and vitamin D and B12, the common nutrients of concern to those who adopt a strictly limited plant-based diet. Dr. Sebi's website mentions that in his products, some ingredients are patented and not specified. This is important, as it is unclear which nutrition you get and how much you get, it make difficult to know if you will fulfill your daily nutrient requirements. Another significant issue with Dr. Sebi's diet policy is the lack of objective evidence to support it, not based on actual research.

He mentions that acid development in your body is regulated by the foods and supplements mentioned in his food. In order to hold PH level of blood between 7.36 and 7.44, the body strictly controls the acid-base balance, naturally rendering the body mildly alkaline. Blood pH will go out of that range in extreme cases, such as ketoacidosis from diabetic conditions. Without instant medical treatment, this can be devastating.

The Sebi plan has no actual evidence to support its arguments, like so many other diet fads (GM diet, here's watching you), Taub-Dix says. Not only diet mainly depend on supplements marketed by the firm, but even names are misleading, as there are currently no credentials or qualifications for Dr. Sebi (whose real name is "Alfredo Bowman") exist.

"Taub-Dix says," I agree that Sebi's name almost gives the diet legitimacy or enables you think it's a reliable diet because he's just not a physician at all. "Another point is that, in case you have advice on what to buy, you need to be aware of every diet where someone sells something to you, such as supplements." Moreover, according to Taub-Dix, the diet's promises of detoxifying and curing the system are deceptive and potentially dangerous. Your liver functions and kidneys are already in very good at eliminating toxins from the body, but there is no evidence that, according to the Mayo Clinic, any foods or drugs can either assist or impede this process.

The key fear of Taub-Dix is that "healing" promises of the plan will lead certain individuals who are treating a disease to follow the diet as a substitute for their drugs that can be harmful. If you're trying to manage a condition, before making significant decisions about your medications or diet, be sure to consult with a doctor.

The doctor Sebi's plan will probably leave you struggling short in terms of your nutrition, especially when proteins are involved. Although the diet allows for nuts and seeds that might have some nutrient content, the total lack of animal foods would likely leave you nutrition-deficient as per Taub-Dix.

Although it may be possible to manage your protein intake on a diet focused on plants, it can be difficult to do so. And the restriction of animal products (such as tofu or vegetarian burgers, for instance) and nutrients outside the diet's own product by the Dr. Sebi diet will make it much harder.

According to H. Chan the School Public Health, on average, a person needs almost 7 g of protein per Twenty pounds of body weight every day. So, you can eat about 56 g of protein daily if you reach 160 pounds. For background, as per the USDA's Food-Data Central, a 1-ounce portion of Sebi-approved walnuts provides just over Four grams of protein. You can also be left lacking in omega-3 fatty acids by limiting animal products, Taub-Dix says. Omega-3s, according to the Penn State Milton S. Hershey Medical Center, are critical for brain function, which contributes to your memory. Deficiency cans results to symptoms such as tiredness, poor memory and dry skin.

Dr. Sebi's diet plan also prevents all processed foods, as per Taub-Dix, which is also not necessarily a positive thing. Generally, super-processed foods do not have significant health benefits, but the processed foods could be part of the safe and balanced diet, such as canned fruit or vegetables. They aren't just convenient, readily accessible and easy to prepare with, making meal preparation even more feasible, but most of these packaged foods are also filled with nutrients that the average person might not have been likely to get from their normal dietary habits, Taub-Dix says.

While the focus of Dr. Sebi's diet on adding plenty of fruit and veggies is undoubtedly a positive feature of an otherwise deficient regimen, Taub-Dix says this is not a diet that will have many advantages. It is not a bad thing to add more whole foods, but it is difficult to get the range of ingredients your body requires because of the excessively stringent nature of this approach.

It is important to prioritize the advice of a health care provider, especially for all those aiming at Dr. Sebi's plan to reduce or alleviate a disease or illness. It is best to consult with a doctor before attempting some kind of diet to make sure it is a good plan for you.

Finally, research has also shown that your food may alter your urine pH slightly and temporarily, but not the pH of the blood. Thus, adopting the diet of Dr. Sebi would not make any difference in the long term.

Chapter 2: Foods recommended by Dr. Sebi.

2.1 List of foods approved by Dr. Sebi (food groups)

The Sebi's Diet is purely based on a vegan diet the program focuses on the whole diet based on plants. It emphasizes foods which have been classified as alkaline by Dr. Sebi. It implies that certain plant-based foods (shown below) are not permitted to be consumed. It is important to be on the authorized food list for all the foods you can eat when following this diet plan. Food list by Dr. Sebi with approved food items is given below.

Vegetables: Asparagus, Cucumbers, Squash, Chickpeas, Amaranth greens, Mushrooms (except Shitake), Onions, Olives, Bell peppers, Amaranth Okra, Avocado, Purslane, atones (cherry and plum only), Dandelion greens Sea vegetables, (Wakame/Dulce/Arame/Hijiki/Nori), Chayote, Tom Tomatillo, Garbanzo beans, Turnip greens Kale, Watercress, Lettuce (except for Iceberg), Wild arugula, Mexican squash, Zucchini.

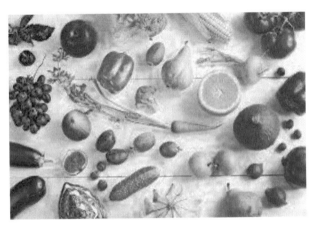

Fruits: Apples, Pears, Figs, Seeded, Cherries, Prunes, Mango, Soft Jelly Coconuts, Cantaloupe, Seeded key limes, Cactus fruit, (Latin or West Indian markets), Papayas, Tamarind, Plums, Seeded grapes, raisins, Bananas, Peaches, Currants, Seeded melons, Oranges, Soursops.

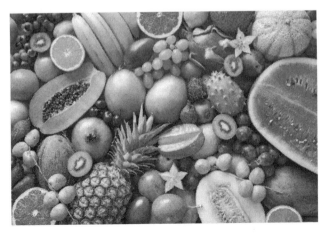

Nuts: Raw Sesame "Tahini" Butter, Brazil nuts, Hemp seed, raw sesame seeds, Walnuts.

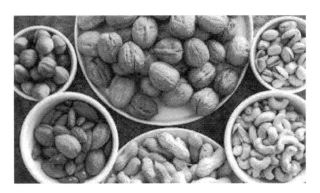

Herb: Achiote, Basil, Onion powder Oregano, Bay leaf, Sage, Habanero Cloves, Sweet basil, Dill, Savory, Cayenne Thyme, Tarragon.

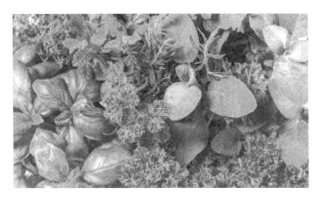

Oils: Hemp seed oil, Avocado oil, Coconut oil (not cooked), Grapeseed oil, Olive oil (not cooked), Sesame oil.

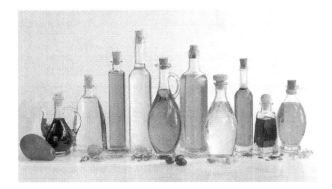

Grains: Amaranth, Rye, Chamomile, Burdock, Ginger, Red raspberry, Quinoa, Wild rice, Herbal teas, Fonio, Spelt, Kamut, Tef Anise, Fennel, Elderberry, Tila, Salt, you may consume the pure sea salt with diet or powdered granulated seaweed.

Sweeteners: Alkaline sweeteners. On this food intake, sugar is not permitted, but some alkaline sugar substitutes are allowed. Date glucose (from dried dates) and natural cactus agave syrup can be eaten.

Non – GMO Foods:

You should concentrate on foods derived from plants that are untreated or minimally processed. Also, the foods ones eat must be non-GMO. Used to prevent pesticides and other additives applied to non-organic foods, it is safer to consume organic-food as much of it as possible. As soon as the foods of preference meet the above requirements, they are likely to eventually allow in diet of Dr. Sebi.

The Doctor Sebi food list was considered by some dieters to be much restrictive for their taste. Nevertheless, faithful adherents of the diet believe that inside the list there are still enough foods to enable you to have a variety. A traditional Dr. Sebi diet menu might look like veggies pan-seared on either a bed of wild rice, in avocado oil, or a broad green salad with a seasoning of olive oil as well as a hint of agave syrup. Although that can take some time to become used to it, the food checklist of Dr. Sebi could be easy to stick to and follow for a healthy diet plan.

2.2. Foods you should never eat (and why)

Below are the main foods items that need to be avoiding when following Dr. Sebi's diet:

All types of meat, fish and seafood, Eggs, Wheat, Dairy products, Fast foods, Sugar, Seedless fruits, Garlic, Corn (and product containing corn), All types food that has been processed, GMO foods, any foods that contains artificial food colors and flavors, foods with preservatives and any type of added vitamins or minerals, Soy, Poultry, all food items that contains yeast and baking powder, Alcohol is strictly prohibited.

As this is a nutritional plan that excludes certain groups of foods, it is essential to use particular nutrients in your diet. Broadly speaking, you might need vitamins including B-12 vitamins, as well as some other vitamins and minerals, like iron, omega-3 fatty acid and calcium, etc. However, you can get plenty of them from plant-based diet if you choose them wisely and consume more than one form of plant origin in a single meal. Or you may order Dr. Sebi items, which had some herbs and minerals that will offer you vitamins that are lacking in your diet, but visit your physician before trying them. The orders can be placed via Amazon.

2.3. List of herbs Doctor Sebi: Green Food plus, Sea Moss, Viento and others.

I love how herbal tea consumption has resulted in my general well-being. They help me retain a well-balanced body and have supported one's body to recover itself. Each body is distinct and different herbs will solve the same problem that you might have in various ways, so I recommend that you should do your own research-work and communicating with an herbalist (who understands the African Bio-Mineral Balance) even if you're an herbal medicine specialist or have a name for a disease. Following are also the plants I like to use for repair, in no precise order.

1. Sea Moss-in conjunction with Bladderwrack, I normally drink it. use hemp milk some dates, and cloves to make a special drink from it. 92 out of 102 minerals composing the human body are found in it. I like it wet. It serves to remind myself to Milo, kind of thing. I prefer to drink it in the morning and in the evening. Also, I utilize it several times per week to cleanse my face. I simply use spring water to incorporate a dime-sized quantity of powder, end up making it like a paste and spread this over my face. Around 5 mins or more, I keep it on, and rinse. * Try regularly our multi-mineral, Cell which helps you, if you don't really like the taste of Sea Moss.

Dr. Sebi also often spoke favorably for sea moss; it's almost a common diet item that is a part of daily life for all of us who adopt his diet. He said that, there is still seems to be uncertainty about it which sort of seaweed (species) are called "Irish moss" and how much nutritional value they have. a "Today, however, Ireland sea moss, nod simple moss may be referred to as a variety of various seaweeds, like (but probably not restricted to) Kappaphycus, Chondrus crispus, alvarezii (a.k.a Eucheuma cottonii) as well as various species inside the genus Gracilaria, based on where you live on the planet.

Gigartinales, Chondrus crispus and cymbopogon alvarezii refer to the same group, but Gracilaria refers to the group of Gracilariales.

K. Alvarezii belongs to a group called Solieriaceae. In contrast, the Chondrus crispus belongs to Gigartinaceae's family, and Gracilaria refers to the group of Gracilariaceae. Seaweed naming convention utilizes the naming system, a "two-term naming scheme."

Knowing this helps to classify the genus to which a certain species belongs, from their name alone. The group to which the species belongs is identified by the first part of its name, whereas the second section describes the species inside the group, i.e. species belongs to the genus Chondrus is Chondrus crispus. In colder waters, Chondrus crispus develops and occurs in excess around the mountainous parts of the Europe's Atlantic coasts, particularly Ireland and the United Kingdom, and Iceland. It can be located on the Canadian and North American Atlantic coasts.

It has a smooth and cartilages consistency in its moist and natural state and it may have different colors from greenish-yellow to red or dark purple to purple-brown. It does have a pale yellow or translucent color when cleaned and sun-dried, which is typically how this will look once you buy the dried plant.

2. Dandelion Root: While I have never been a real hardcore coffee addict, I prepare Dandelion Root Tea that tastes quite like coffee whenever I want to feel the flavor. Introduce Hemp-Milk with Date Syrup and then you've created a latte for yourself. What's really incredible about it, this is also a liver cleanser. Cleaning up the liver offers you some vitality in return. So, consuming this in morning is indeed a perfect substitute for coffee and helps the body to stay in detox mode rather than having all the acid with in the body which coffee drinking can generate.

3. Damiana: I drink Damiana whenever I feel mentally unbalanced, anxious or nervous. Even though it is marketed as an herbal remedy, it helps me feel relaxed and not excited. Still, the experience might be unique for others. A perfect tea when you're having menstruation. Try Nerves Support in-case you are searching for a treatment that can assist you with anxiety and depression.

4-5 Burdock Root and Combo Sarsaparilla-Burdock Root contains up to 102 minerals at low concentrations in the body. To offer me a mineral boost, I want to mix this with other herbs. Because Sarsaparilla contains the highest amount of iron and works as a magnet for minerals, I always combine them (usually, like Linden Flower, with a third herb that rounds out the flavor).

6. Yellow Dock: I introduce this to the tea combos when my skin may feel out of whack, indicating my lymphatic system feels overwhelmed or I have a rash with something I have affected (or touched me). It doesn't always taste fine on its own. I even grind it up and prepare a face mask out of it in a coffee grinder (adding it mainly to Sea Moss).

7. Blue Vervain: When I feel lacking in magnesium, I drink this. Indications of this are that my brain is overdriving to one problem, and I cannot "wind it off" or I cannot sleep. That relieves anxiety. I typically take-out supplement for Nerve-Support in capsule form, since it tastes like a metallic chemical that's not perfect. But I can mix it with Damiana or Linden as a tea that has a light floral taste. * Aside-MANY people who routinely smoke marijuana are seriously deficient in magnesium.

8. Cascara Sagrada: - This is what I call 'Boo Boo Tea,' lmao. I go straight for this, if I'm constipated. It also doesn't taste amazing, but I equate this to brown alcohol. I often get a couple of shots. I recommend drinking it at night, so I'll be ready to go in the morning. I do not recommend drinking it and then moving out for a long period where you'll have to use a toilet in someone else's home. If so, I would suggest covering the smell from some of the Bathroom Drops,

particularly if you consumed some junk in the first place to become constipated.

9. Elderberry: When I have been around sick people, and I'd like to give some boost to immunity, Elderberry pushes my immune system in hyperdrive. But be careful. You can get extremely nauseous when you eat too much Elderberry. Also-to get them more appealing, a perfect complement to other herbs.

10. Linden Flower: These are perfect for lung mucus expulsion. Truly calming. When we feel dry throat or a constant cough, it's my time to go. It has a floral taste that is mild. Great compliment to herbal extracts with strong flavors to round out.

11. BLACK WALNUT: Normally used to treat parasitic worms, like diphtheria and syphilis, and certain other diseases. It is used for leukemia as well. Some individuals use Black Walnut mostly as gargle, apply this as a hair dye into the scalp, or place this on skin in order to treat wounds.

12. Chickweed: use this thing for constipation, stomach & bowel issues and blood disorders along with asthma and other lung-related diseases. It can be used for scurvy and psoriasis as well as scratching, and muscle & joint pain as an enzyme inhibitor. For skin conditions, including boils, sores and ulcers, it can be applied to the skin.

13. NETTLE: is used for hair growth stimulation. In individuals with diabetes, it helps regulate blood sugar. It decreases gingivitis-related bleeding, treats kidney and helps in recovering urinary tract disorders, and offers water retention. It prevents and handles diarrhea.

14. Mugwort: To induce digestive juices and bile secretion, mugwort is used. It is frequently used to prevent digestive tract diseases and to help with all digestive system issues and is said to have an anti-fungal effect. It has antibacterial, expectorative and antiasthmatic properties. It can be used in the treatment of a wide range of infectious diseases, like tapeworm, roundworm, and thread-worm. Mugwort is thought to be successful. For irregular cycles and other menstrual issues, females take mugwort. It is sometimes used as a tonic for the liver; for circulation promotion; and as a sedative. If pregnant, do not use) *.

15. Sage: For digestive issues, including lack of appetite, gas, stomach pain, diarrhea, bloating, and heartburn, SAGE can be used. It can also be used for minimizing transpiration & saliva increased production; for depression, memory loss & Alzheimer's disease. It has been used by women for painful menstrual cycles, to fix irregular milk flow during breastfeeding, and to minimize menopausal hot flashes.

16. Sarsaparilla: For the prevention of gout, gonorrhea, open sores, rheumatoid arthritis, pain in

joints, cough, fever, high blood pressure, skin diseases, and indigestion, sarsaparilla is considered effective. It also has the maximum (according to Dr. Sebi) iron content of any herb.

17. Strawberry leaf: The main use of Strawberries Leaves is to alleviate gastrointestinal discomfort and joint pain. They include essential minerals, such as iron, an important component of production of red blood cells, and hemoglobin, which helps to support anemia. It helps in reducing high blood pressure due to its vasodilating effects. It is also advertised as a blood purifier and provides relief from mucus.

18. Bladderwrack: is a type of kelp which is used as a therapeutic strategy for obesity and cellulite to activate the thyroid gland. It is rich in iodine and helps to improve the metabolism. It also decreases inflammation, improves muscles, enhances circulation, it protects the skin, supports vision, and prevents premature ageing; also it reduces cancer risk, and improves heart health.

In your search for a healthy body, I hope the list provided above will helps you. It's a recommendation I want to make to take each herb one at a time and to learn how each one makes you feel personally. Reading books and listening to people is fine, but finding it out by yourself helps you with a more intimate view about what is good for you.

2.4. The shopping list of Doctor Sebi's approved products

So, you've got Dr. Sebi's Dietary Guidance on board, and you're happy to shop? Few things are fairly easy to locate, but you will have to look a little harder for few others. You will have to search beyond the model you're used to for conventional food stores or the big box stores whether you're searching for organic or herbal goods or grains.

Taking the bananas that are approved, such as orange, burro, and baby bananas. You might buy one of these in a normal grocery shop, and you'll notice a bunch more of what you need for this Serbian diet plan if you search a little deeper.

Vegetables: According to Dr. Sebi "Never use the microwave, this will kill all your food."

Amaranth greens, Bell Peppers, a variety of Spinach, Dandelion greens, Cucumber, Avocado, Burro Banana, Asparagus, Chayote (Mexican Squash), Jicama, Garbanzo beans (chickpeas), Izote "cactus flower/ cactus leaf," Kale, Lettuce (all, but not Iceberg), Mushrooms (all, but not Shitake), Mustard greens, Olives, Onions, Okra, Squash, Nopales (Mexican Cactus), Poke salad –greens, Spinach (use sparingly), String beans, Tomato –only cherry and plum, Tomatillo, Turnip greens,

Zucchini, Sea Vegetables (dulse / wakame /arame/ nori/ hijiki).

Fruits: "No canned and seedless fruits". Dr. Sebi.

Apples, Bananas (only the smallest one are allowed or the Burro (mid-size original banana), Berries complete variety Elderberries in any form (but no cranberries), Cherries, Currants, Figs, Dates, Grapes –seeded, Cantaloupe, Mango, Limes, Orange, Melons, Peaches, Pears, Plums, Prunes, Papayas, Raisins –seeded, Soft Jelly Coconuts, Soursops, Sugar apples- chermoya.

Herbal Teas: Alvaca, Chamomile, Anise, Cloves, Ginger, Lemongrass, Red Raspberry, Sea Moss Tea, Fennel

Spices & Seasonings: Mild Flavors, Bay leaf, Cilantro, Basil, Marjoram, Oregano, Tarragon, Sweet Basil, Thyme, Achiote, Cayenne, Cumin, Coriander, Onion Powder, Sage, Dill, Salty Flavors, Pure Sea Salt, Powdered Granulated Seaweed, Kelp/Dulce.

Sweet Flavors: Pure Maple Syrup only B grade is recommended, Maple "Sugar" (derived from maple syrup), Date "Sugar" (derived from dates), Pure Agave Syrup derived from cactus.

Nuts & Seeds: Raw Almonds, Almond Butter, Raw Sesame, Raw Sesame Seeds, "Tahini" Butter, and Walnuts/Hazelnut.

It is surprising that people have "allergies with wheat", reason behind it's not a natural grain; it is produced by science and is a hybrid product, and it is acid-based.

Natural Growing Grains have a nature of alkaline-based foods; it is therefore recommended that you must use the following products instead of Wheat:

Black Rice, Amaranth, Quinoa, Rye, Spelt, Tef, Wild Rice, Kamut.

Chapter 3: Dr. Sebi's diet for management of various diseases

3.1. Dr. Sebi's diet with diabetes and herpes

Dr. Sebi's remedy to cure Diabetes is straightforward and needs to have very little money, but few will obey his plan. His idea was quite easy. Only stop eating.

Many people tend to get their foot chopped off before they even have to stop eating. Yet in 27 days during fasting, Dr. Sebi healed his own diabetes. Remember we discuss in the introduction that Sebi was a self-educated man and he was diagnosed with diabetes.

Many people have also published the same findings. One person on You-Tube also confirmed that he successfully treated his diabetes by following Dr. Sebi's fasting program.

Dr. Sebi stated, "Mucus is really the source of all types of disease, and mucus falls only after you've absorbed anything that shouldn't have in your bloodstream."

Dr. Sebi's strategy is to rid the body of needless mucosa, which is considered the origin of all diseases. He states this: "Our study indicates that any type of disorder has its origin when mucous membrane becomes weakened. i.e. whether there is excess mucous inside the bronchial tubes, the resulting disease will relates to bronchitis; if it is found in inside the lungs, the resultant disease will be known as pneumonia; and inside pancreatic duct, the resultant issue will simply be diabetes; mucous in the joints called arthritis.

Besides, the mucosa in the retina causes blindness; if observed across the thyroid gland, the same will result in thyroid cancer. Basically, the illness will occur in the body whenever this stagnant poison is build up in the body.

The healing diet can be found mentioned below it's important to remember that Sebi has suggested foods mentioned here for recovery from a disease for more than 30 years. Suppose your favorite food is absent from our list. In that case, we assure you that based on our research and findings, it has little nutritious benefit and could be harmful to your health; that is the reason we have neglected that and not included in our list of approved food items.

So, what if you have MUCUS build up in your body?

If you do have diabetes, you might've got mucus in the pancreatic duct. Thus, part of the procedure (fasting) is to eliminate the mucus. His mother took 57 days of fasting to clear the mucus. For this moment, Dr. Sebi must have kept her peaceful and quiet. I fasted on four different occasions, most of which were 12 days, and then on my last fast, I saw no mucus at all.

The really nice herbal tea for mucus that I created is Elderberry tea, The Red Raspberry and Black Walnut Leaves or Burdock. Take a full tablespoon of every herb and put them all in one & half liters of fresh spring water and wait to boil the water. Boil the herbal tea for about 15 minutes, and then include another half-liter of water. Get the herbal tea to another boil again and then remove from stove. Strain all the herbs and set all of them aside for use for upcoming days. On next day, you can reuse the extracted herbs again. You may put the herbal tea in carafe or you may store it inside the refrigerator so that it may be consumed later on. Drink the tea for whole day as required.

Besides fasting, you need to continue with Dr. Sebi Verified Diet Schedule and monitor your diet closely. There are many other things you must care for that will help with diabetes, too.

Mulberry-Leaves and Black-Seeds are the most recommended replacements. Black Seeds have been studied and proven that only little amount of them let say only 2 teaspoons in single day is enough to cure diabetes.

Figleaves are known as the best-selling leaf today in the market commonly used for curing diabetes according to a survey published in 1998. Mulberry leaves are also the number one treatment used by diabetic patients in the Middle East. You can simply add some black seeds to your herbal teas too.

Some useful items are Swiss chard, Sour melon, Garlic, avocado, Okra, Ginseng, Fenugreek and Red Clover.

3.2. Herpes

Having a series of fasting or consuming food items that are much less toxic to the electrical body would undoubtedly aim to rid everyone of herpes. The purpose is to build an atmosphere in which the cause of the disease cannot survive. Your cells are in search of oxygen. Toxins such as medicines for herpes will steal the oxygen from cells, which, in most instances, will tie with herpes.

Healing herpes is going to be taking some cleaning and plant-based Iron products. Implement the same way we are doing to cure HIV. You're going to start with Iron Plus with Bio Ferro.

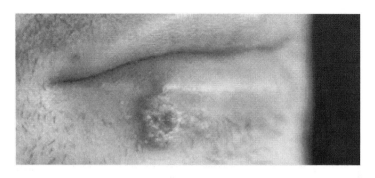

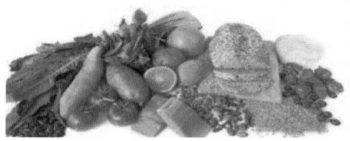

Plus Powder (Bromide for tea)

The key to success is NUTRITION. Although the immune response is getting Support from iron, much of the mineral nutrients required will come from bromide plus powder; you just have to make the tea then drink it. Boil some water, pour into a small blender, turn it on, introduce about one teaspoon of bromide, and let it mix for a couple of minutes. Do so twice or more than once a day.

A perhaps a more significant way of treating herpes is dealing with foods that you shouldn't bring in your mouth and the body. Stay out of the starches and sweets. Very minimal portions of fruit or vegetable food are sweet. Have more bitter food than sweet food. However, there is a lot of lettuce to choose from, however. For healing reasons but stay away from avocados and chickpeas, avoid quinoa and gravitate and move towards more zucchini, use squash, cactus flower or leaf.

If you already have plant-based iron green tea such as the burdock, the dandelion, the yellow dock, that will surely help. Consume as many days as you are able to; a minimum of ten days. You don't have to mix it. That's your choice if you want to. Depending upon where you are, they can be challenging to locate. You might need to order these roots through online herbal websites. (Already mentioned in the previous section).

Practice fasting; prepare to get on with it. The more fasting you have, the more chances of healing you will have.

If you're feeling weak, eat some dates. They're sweet, but they're not supposed to agitate your cells. Eat just when you are weak.

You may have salads just like you were enjoying a bag full of potato chips. Get a crisp light (but no iceberg lettuce). The response to what Sebi tries to teach us is to get rid of mucus build up in the body, and it ends up going like this:

There is just one disorder, and this is the product of the mucous membrane being damaged. The mucous membrane is important to preserve health as it is that membrane which covers the cells. If you tear down the mucous layer, it transforms into pus and reveals the cells.

i.e., Sickle Cell Anemia happens when blood plasma is broken and turns to sickle by a mucous membrane. The mucus falls in the plasma and into the cell itself, splits and dis-unifies the cell. By removing the mucous, the cell get unites again. You need to feed a patient with massive amounts of iron phosphate to sustain that amount. Not iron oxide.

Iron-based herbal substances developed by Dr. Sebi, like Iron Plus or Bio Ferro, supply the body from over 14 primary organic (carbon-hydrogen-oxygen) plants and herbal minerals.

A collection of vegetation cell-based food items includes Iron Phosphate, but are extracted from electrically activated tropical plants; some originate from tropical Africa and Honduras. Also, some belong to the Caribbean; others might be from Latin American countries.

Herbal plants in Dr. Sebi's vegetation-based cell food are strongly electrical. Their molecular structures are complete, and it's based on carbon. They would quickly assimilate and energies the human body with foods served by nature to us. The nutrients provide your body with the requisite phosphates and carbonates along with iodides and bromide ... also called the food of life!

3.3. Liver cleansing with the diet of Dr. Sebi

You may have read of allopathic medications' adverse effects because most of them are moderate acne, digestive problems or nausea, right? Several researchers have eventually demonstrated that consuming so many allopathic medications clearly influences the kidneys and liver. Now, you're also supposed to think beyond acne and nausea problems, and this isn't all the allopathic drugs that can do with you. If you depend on unnecessary drugs, you are at risk. Various variables lead to this durability. But even though you realize that your liver is in trouble because of the fast cure medications that you take, you're always doing the same thing; you're certainly at fault. This implies that you don't even trust your long-term wellbeing. We're going to look at Sebi's liver disease treatment kit and its advantages, but before going for that, let me remind you one thing most of you are reading this book because of allopathic medications. These medications, which we also term modern medicine, have rendered Dr. Sebi's cure kit for the liver necessary for about all. In simple words, you'll see why and how to see some of the components in Sebi's liver disease cure package.

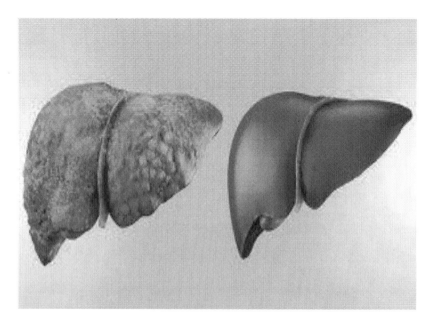

Sebi's Liver Diseases Treatment Kit includes:

Punarnavadi Mandoor: It is a combination of Punarnava and many other herbs, which have hepatoprotective nature. The first component in Dr. Sebi's liver disorder cure package is a blend of up to one dozen herbs. Both these herbs are obtained from their native lands.

Sutsekhar Ras Gold: It is a Fine powder of Shuddha Parada (known as Herbal distilled Mercury). Swarna Bhasma, (known as Bhasma of Gold), Tankana Bhasma (called Borax), The Tamra Bhasma (It is prepared from Copper), The Gandhaka (you may call it Purified and processed Sulphur), Shuddha Vatsanabha (maybe known as Purified Aconitum Ferox), and Shankha Bhasma (It is a Conch Shell which is processed, purified and combined to make Sutshekhar ras gold. These things are known as the ashes of metals that are purified to make Sure that these strong metals may only contain the healing properties in them.

Chandrakala Ras: It is another herbal formula that is a natural combination of uncommon herbs and solid minerals. Ela (Cardamom), Amla, Camphor, Jatiphala, and Shalmali are among the well-known herbal ingredients for Chandrakanta-ras. So, this herbal combination is required if you want to maintain the liver intact.

Punarnava Herbal blend: Since the punarnava is among the best herbs that we have for curing liver problems, Sebi wants to use it against all liver diseases. Also, to improve the overall health of the liver in particular. These ingredients used in it are a blend of many herbs. These herbs used here will differ based on different liver disorders you may be suffering from.

Sarphunka Plant: This is known as a plant's scientific name, and Dr. Sebi used it to cope with multiple liver disorders. Not just that, it holds a unique spot in Ayurveda's ancient healing science. Because of its unmatched role in curing liver disease, that is included in Dr. Sebi's liver disease cure kit.

AHP Zinc Powder: Liver probably is the most essential organ in the human body. Liver contains too many enzymes and hormones along with components that are essential for our body to perform many functions. It detoxifies different metabolites and generates enzymes, produces synthesizes proteins, and makes the biochemicals required for digestion. These are only few of the liver's activities, and, besides, they have an indirect effect on human well-being when they involve the operation of the digestive tract and the gall bladder. Since the liver has too many irreplaceable functions, and too many other body organs are directly based on it, you mustn't neglect it anymore. The first most thing you can do if you frequently consume antibiotics and allopathic medicines for any reason, make sure to get your liver screened. If you've already completed the test and, sadly, there are any complications, you can just order Dr. Sebi's liver disorder cure package. You can buy all the kits online by searching on Google or follow "drsebihealing.com."

Benefits of Dr. Sebi Package for Curing Liver disease.

There are so many liver diseases cured using Dr. Sebi's liver disease cure package. For example, the following liver diseases are causing problems for millions of human beings. Luckily, we can easily get rid of them by using just the herbal solution provided by Dr. Sebi. The following are the main issues cured by using Dr. Sebi's Kit for Liver diseases.

- Cancer of the liver

- Liver with fat on it

- Hepatitis A, Hepatitis B, and Hepatitis C

- Cirrhosis of liver

- Diseases across the Gall's bladder

- Pancreas-related disorders

These issues and several other health problems may be resolved by using Dr. Sebi's liver disorder cure kit, and they are closely linked to the Liver. Besides, the toxicity introduced by improper usage of allopathic medications may also be reduced. And it just costs $160 to allow the use of all these opportunities. Yes, in just $160, you can get a complete and comprehensive solution against all the major liver problems. Besides the herbs and other herbal mixtures, which are recommended by Dr. Sebi, you may get a plan to alter your diet plan and lifestyle. Dr. Sebi has always believed in keeping the food safe for the body.

So, with Sebi's kit for curing your liver, you'll even get clear guidance about how you may use it and any other improvements you need to make in your lifestyle to hold your liver condition in control. You can place an order for your pack from "drsebihealing.com" now. Please notice that Dr. Sebi's liver cure kit would last for only two months, so this is probably the lowest time required by your liver to use these herbal medicines kit. Also, unlike the other Sebi's kits, you may customize the kit according to your liver problem. Upon your check-out process, you will then be required to provide some basic information regarding your disease along with the issues you face. Herbal doctors will tailor the Sebi's liver disease care package specifically for your body and its issues.

3.4. The best electric foods and herbs Dr. Sebi for hypertension

When walls of the vessels are crossed, or plaqued and get stuffed, the blood flow is reduced when it flows from the heart towards the aorta; hence pressure is produced by the arteries; hence blood pressure rises and becomes greater than normal above the point typically meant to be, the resulting consequence is, hypertension (also known high blood pressure) has formed.

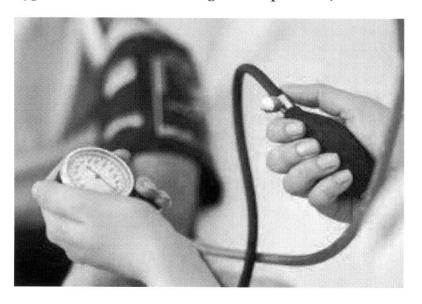

Diet is at the top when it comes to the causes of high blood pressure, particularly in the United States. It has been reported in a study that over 85% of cases of high blood pressure are directly linked to bad dieting habits. In every age group and gender, African Americans are reported to have more cases of high blood pressure than other US races. High blood pressure may result in other diseases like strokes, large heart than normal, artery coronary diseases, typhoid fever, tonsillitis, scarlet fever, and often kidney diseases. These diseases are likely to have high blood pressure (known as hypertension, too) among Afro-Americans.

3.5. What is considered as a high blood pressure situation?

Suppose you want to measure the blood pressure. In that case, all you need is a tool called blood pressure gauge or B.P apparatus, which is also called a sphygmomanometer which is capable of recording two types of information regarding Blood Pressure: the 1st one is known as the systolic, it is the higher reading whereas 2nd one is known as the diastolic, and is considered as lower reading.

Therefore, diastolic may be considered less problematic than systolic elevated blood pressure readings since systolic unveils the pressure built up by blood when it is pumped from the heart towards the aorta right before it passes into the passageways inside the arteries. When the systolic reading becomes high, blood pressure is deemed high. Also, the arteries' walls become clogged and there become plaques inside the walls that impede blood flow. Under normal situations, the reading of systolic high blood pressure ranges from 120-150 millimeters. On the other hand, a high reading, let say 140/190, points towards high blood pressure and any reading over 180/115, maybe even more.

What are the causes of high blood pressure?

High blood pressure situations are induced by consuming food that creates plaque that clogs around the arteries' wall while the blood circulating inside the arteries is high, thereby causing increased pressure inside the arteries throughout the circulation process. From the heart to other body organs, the blood flows directly from the heart towards the aorta and arteries. The blood supply in the arteries' corridors is suppressed when walls of the arteries become narrow, and they get hardened due to heavy plaque-induced by poor dieting.

Another thing to keep up in mind is that when a person's age is increased, the arteries automatically get hardened because many times the diet is poor. When people get older, this triples the risk of triggering and causing high blood pressure.

High blood pressure is caused by:

Apart from the hardening and clogging of arteries owing to the inadequate blood supply, which may cause elevated blood pressure. Synthetic medications, fatty foods, and harmful patterns of behavior trigger elevated blood pressure: the following are also cases of high blood pressure.

Stress, Tobacco, Aging, Bad diet is also a very important cause: many coffees, Fried and oily foods items and other processed foods and Overeating.

High blood pressure Symptoms:

Dr. Sebi' sees the effects of high blood pressure as the "navy seal sniper attacker," and there are hardly any visible indicators of high blood pressure. This does not indicate, though, that there are no complications. The only visible signs of high blood pressure are difficulty in breathing; the eyes can get distorted; a headache can arise?

A person claimed that one of his aunts had elevated blood pressure. Her blood pressure signs were dizziness and that her heartbeat was fasting. "But, because signs of high blood pressure are not often apparent, it received a reputation as the" sniper killer of the navy seal.

Dr. Sebi's recommended diet for curing High blood pressure:

"All the elevated blood pressure medications imitate water; hence it's a common-sense that you ought to consume plenty of freshwaters," hence you need to consume pure spring water.

Low blood pressure medicine causes thinning of the blood, so that drinking water thins the blood. Divide the weight by 2, so consume the sum of ounces of water. For starters, you'd break 150/2, which is 75 ounces of water a day, if you weigh 150.

Eating five separate kinds of fruits and vegetables in a day will help avoid clogging of the arteries and help to avoid shut down of artery walls and of plaque deposits. Asparagus, broccoli, onions, seeded grapes, oranges, and peaches are some common fruits and vegetables rich in antioxidants that help resist artery walls and plaques; you may see the diet guide for more help on natural fruits and veggies to cure high blood pressure.

Potassium-rich diets are helpful since potassium encourages the body to release sodium to cope with high blood pressure issues. Eat mostly potassium-rich fruits and vegetables like small red-potatoes, whereas stop salty foods. See the dietary guide for more details, as mentioned above.

Fruits and vegetables rich in fiber are good for curing high blood pressure; as they can relieve pressure, which helps to eliminate waste that has been sucked around the artery walls.

High blood pressure may be experienced after eating:

Most of the cases of High blood pressure are recorded after eating. It is critical because after you have eaten something, it is difficult to know its causes. You need to recognize what things to eliminate that could be dangerous to increasing your blood pressure. These are lethal to your good health but what you should not consume is as important as what you should consume. When eating, you do not want to get elevated blood pressure. Stop the following foods:

Particularly if the meal is called a nutritious meal, stop overheating.

Don't consume a salty meal, but keep clear of the salt. Inside the walls of arteries, salt transforms and activates plaque. In general, these foods include salt, but please read the label placed on foods you consume to prevent sodium intake: avoid soda, baking soda, soy sauce, meat tenderizers, and monosodium glutamate (MSG).

Lots of meat, candy, baked products, and cakes. Stop them all. Don't buy any frozen goods, which stands with fruits and vegetables, making sure you don't buy canned food. Eat nothing produced with milk, really rich in salt, and no cheese at all, yogurt, and alcohol are prohibited. Take out dairy items from your diet. Do not eat very late in the evening,

Do not consume rice. Instead, eat brown and wild rice in case you do so.

3.6. Dr. Sebi's recommended food for curing Hypertension

Dr. Sebi proposes the following herbs as they open up the blood vessels and arteries' wall and remove plaques from the artery wall. These herbs rich in minerals are organic electric herbs of alkaline origin. They have been investigated and have proved to be great sources of treatment for hypertension. Herbal herbs are typically strong in strength, so much of them for the blood would be heavy in strength. Here is the list:

- Black cohosh

- Basil

- Yellow dock

- Cayenne

- Oregano

- Fennel

Encouragement:

Anyone can overcome hypertension, so as you too. People who have achieved these easy tasks prevail no high blood pressure, and so you will. Now, as you are ready to fight and win with the details provided here. Notice that you can consume a balanced diet with the prescribed fruits, nuts, herb and grains to monitor the rise in blood pressure daily. See the Dietary Guide. Finally, to preserve the weight workout regularly.

3.7. How to lose weight by following your diet

Condition like Overweight and having obesity are characterized as the accumulation of abnormal or unnecessary fat that poses a health danger. The body to mass index or (BMI), is called the weight of an individual (in kgs) divided by square of height (in meters), is a crude population obesity metric. Generally, a person having a BMI of 30 or above is deemed obese. It is deemed overweight by an individual with a BMI equal to or greater than 25.

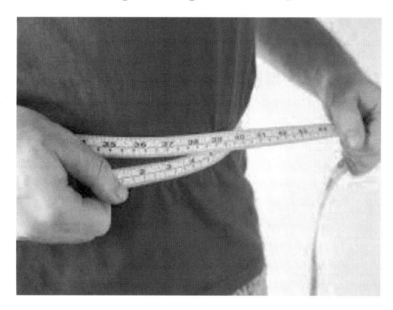

Overweight and obesity significantly contribute to diabetes, coronary disorders and cancer, and a variety of chronic diseases. But being overweight and having obesity were once considered a concern only for countries with high-income. Still, now it's rising significantly in low or middle-income countries, especially urban ones.

Dr. Sebi's diet discourages the Western lifestyle, which is rich in highly processed foods filled with salt, fat, sugar, and calories. Dr. Sebi encourages an unprocessed diet plan instead of processed foods. Many that adopt a plant-based diet appear to have a lower incidence of obesity and cardiac disease than the Western diet.

A 12-month survey of 65 individuals showed that those who adopted an unrestricted, low fat, plant-based, whole-food diet lost dramatically more weight than those who did not adopt the diet. Those on Sebi's diet lost, on average about 26.6 pound (12.1 kgs) at the six-month point, compared to 3.5 pounds or (1.6 kgs) in the controlled community.

Furthermore, except for almonds, beans, avocados, and oils, most items in this diet are poor in calories. Consequently, even though you consume a significant amount of permitted items, it is impossible that this will result in calorie imbalance and contribute to weight gain.

Nevertheless, quite-low-calorie diets will typically not be managed in the long run. When they restore a regular eating schedule, most individuals who adopt these diets recover weight. Since amounts and portions are not defined by this diet, it is impossible to tell if it would supply sufficient calories for effective weight loss.

When adopting the diet or Sebi's menu, weight loss is expected to experience since the Sebi's diet is comprised of raw vegetables, fruits, wheat, nuts, and legumes.

It removes waste, sugar, poultry, and packaged foods, meaning you'll lose weight naturally. Dr. Sebi's diet works like a cleanser food and reaps several rewards, like your body praising you. It is also necessary, regularly, to drink a lot of water. This facilitates the separation from the body of the dangerous components. When this is the aim, it will help you achieve positive results during your journey towards weight loss.

One should consume about 1 gallon of pure water every day, according to Sebi. Do not drink tap water: always ensure that water you drink is 100% pure and clean.

3.8. How to reduce stress and increase cardiac function

Are you familiar with anxiety issues that impact over 18 percent of Americans? About 40 million citizens! This is more than 40 million! The proportion of youth is up to 25 percent. More than 284 million people around the world are impacted. Try to learn the ways through which we can take care of yourself and your health.

Stress and anxiety may contribute to a variety of health complications and mental health disorders. To avoid escalation, side effects and long-term effects, it's also necessary to treat anxiety as it arises. Although western healthcare practices rely on psychiatric care and medical intervention; several simple and easy methods prevent the risks related to anxiety and stress that can easily be adapted to overcome the issues.

Consequences of anxiety and stress and how to avoid:

The long-term impacts of anxiety may be severe; hence anxiety must be treated early and regularly so that serious harmful effects can be avoided and minimized. To stop the risks of fear and fatigue, adopt these basic tips:

1) Have some time for yourself because it is necessary. Life in modern society is too busy that we must calm down and relax occasionally. It is important to take some time to rest and get away from work to cope with chronic stress or anxiety. When the day ends, take some rest and enjoy a sample of Dr. Sebi's Tension Reliever Herbal tea, and spend some time with those you love most.

2) Manage time for those things which bring leisure to your life. Situations in which you do the only job, and no play must be avoided! Give yourself time for stuff you like. Do something that would help you feel comfortable every day so that the tension is eased. It doesn't mean to have tones of time — even fifteen to twenty minutes are enough.

3) One of the easiest methods of relaxing the body and mind is to do some exercise daily. This doesn't mean to be a strenuous activity, so it will enormously boost the mood by enjoying a walk after having your meals or resting before bed.

4) Stress can manage to take a toll on your normal defenses of the body. But having right diet can provide relaxation when consuming the right nutrients. Often the burden of everyday life is natural to feel wrung out. Sadly, we prefer to search for fast food, but do you know high-calorie or sugary snacks just trick us into believing that we feel stronger. Eating nutritious food will potentially give a serious stress reduction and make it a deliberate decision. Follow the Dietary Guide of Sebi and hydrate yourself properly to ensure that you have the right resources for your body to handle everything that comes to your way!

5) Breathing is considered a natural corporal feature and is taken for granted by most people. Stress, however, may cause individuals to slip into a dangerous pattern of breathing and fear. Generally, nervous people take quick, fast breaths at a rising pace. Although this is an indication of fear, it is, in reality, still a source that reinforces the sense of anxiety more. Anxiety contributes to shallow respiration, which contributes to further anxiety, contributing to shallower respiration, etc. As you can expect, everybody believes that building healthy breathing patterns is important and mentioned below are some of the major health advantages of deep breathing techniques:

- Decreases your heart rate

- Control blood pressure

- Decrease build-up of lactic acid

- Core muscle stability is improved

- Decreases adverse effects of cortisol

- Immune system is boosted

- Volume of oxygen is increased being received by body

- Energy metabolism is increased

- Soothing effect on the brain

- Healing capabilities are improved

- Impacts positively on memory

- Improves capabilities for intense exercise.

- Electrical patterns are more organized in the brain

- Honor your heart just as nature demands

On average, a normal heart beats up to 42 million times during a year, pumping blood and creating an electromagnetic field that is detectable from 10 feet away. Unfortunately, the major cause of mortality in the US is heart disease; almost half of adults have cardiovascular complaints. But, remember, the heart is not just a pump, it is associated to love as well. So, think how much your heart is healthy?

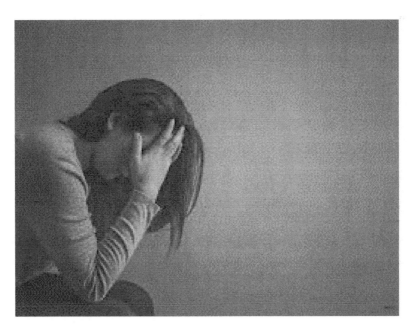

Pressure built-up

Heart failure is triggered by congestion in the circulatory system. Blood arteries lose their resilience and cannot improve the heart's beating operation with their actual elasticity. Sugars and fats that are unsafe render them stiff and limit flow.

Blood pressure is increased by rigidity, causing the heart to work faster to force blood into the tissues. In this closed structure, mucus causes more pressure, putting more stress on the heart during pumping and lungs. Imagine pumping to dense pipe glue instead of liquid around the heating system. There's something about to blast!

Re-Engineering the Heart's Health

Before Sebi took decisive steps to resolve his health issues, he was really poor. He started consuming his native food and developed diabetes, hypertension, impotence, schizophrenia, and hysteria. It was the influence of diet and herbs that spared his life because medical technology did not save him. "The herbs are working for me," said Dr. Sebi, "and I realize I'm satisfied at 82."

Eating any food out of line with the cell predisposition induces illness. Impotence is an early warning indicator that the supply of blood is compromised. Luckily, enriching your body with blessings of nature restores wellness to every aspect of the body as well as mind.

Nourish your Heart

Addressing the dietary requirements of 'healthy' fats along with antioxidants found in nuts and seeds may be one of the easiest approaches to encourage cardiovascular health: consider consuming the following

- Reduces disease risk by using walnuts that contain alpha-linolenic acid.

- Brazil nuts have selenium that restores the equilibrium of fatty acids.

- Hemp seeds keep the blood vessels elastic and dilated.

- Sesame seed decreases cholesterol and eliminates inflammation.

Take diligent care of the cardiovascular function through diet, activity, and mind. A gentle, fun workout makes the core muscle healthy. Maintaining a balanced bodyweight and consuming food prevents the blood from circulating. Maintaining a good outlook promotes long-term well-being. Eat a nutritional diet given Sebi's Nutritional Guide. There are so many things you should do to hold the heart safe for a million more beats! Do you have heart disease following natural solutions.

Mother Nature offers all required essentials to restore dietary destruction and to clear up clogged arteries. When your heart wants extra help, Dr. Sebi's Green Food can softly put your heart muscle back into harmony. Cardiac-healthy herbs recommended by Dr. Sebi's Green Food dramatically improve the heart's health:

Bladderwrack eliminates the fatty deposits that clogged blood arteries.

Tila promotes relaxing, decreases inflammation and lowers blood pressure.

Nettle decreases blood glucose and blood pressure and reduces the chance of illness.

Nopal strengthens the nerves, decreases cholesterol and decreases blood sugar.

Dr. Sebi has also created herbal packets that contain the Lily of the Valley. It is a sweet-smelling plant and produces 40 different cardiac-glycosides that adjust fluid balance; boost contraction strength; restore heartbeat frequency, and overcome valve abnormalities.

Time to Change

Dr. Sebi has always been persistent in finding out the link between mental and physical healing. Dr. Sebi stated, "One of the elements that are so essential for this path to be recognized and understood is the LOVE, yet this was not the term itself. It's the electrical contact between you and any other guy or someone else besides you.

The electromagnetic fields of the hearts are built to bind us. It's beneficial to extend love and goodness. Translating passion into motion produces heartfelt echo and slavery. The basic act of smiling conveys optimistic feelings and awakens affection in the heart. Let's be heart-free, nutritiously free, and electromagnetically linked together.

Whatever you want to do, note that managing persistent stress and anxiety is just as vital to health as any other step you take.

Chapter 4. Dr. Sebi Soups Recipes

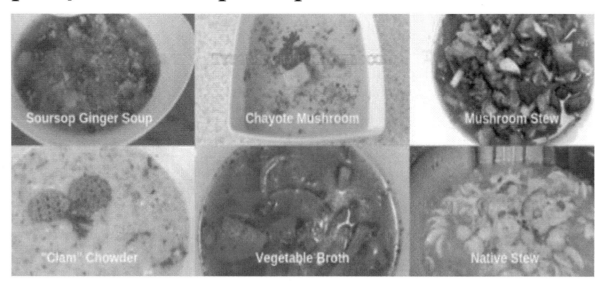

4.1. Dr. Sebi's" cleansing green soup

Serving: 4

Total Time: 1 hour

Ingredients:

- 3 if medium otherwise 2 large onions (yellow color), peeled and chopped them roughly.

- Zucchini 1, washed not peeled, and chopped roughly.

- Dandelion greens 1 bunch.

- Wild arugula1 bunch

- Vegetable broth homemade 4 cups (make it with approved vegetables only)

- Packed basil1/2 cup

- Packed dill1/2 cup

- key lime Juice of 1

- grapeseed oil 3 tbs

- sea salt 1/4 tbs

- avocado1/4

- Cayenne pepper, as per your taste

Directions:

To make this cleaning soup, begin to heat the grapeseed oil in a wide pot on medium-high heat. Add the onion and then cook for 5 mins, stirring regularly, until translucent.

Add the dandelion greens, the zucchini and the wild arugula and simmer for another 5 minutes. Put in vegetable stock (homemade) and wait for a boil, decrease heat and let it cook, cover, for 15-20 minutes. Let it cool, with lid off, for 15 minutes.

If required, combine batches of basil, dill, avocado, lime, sea salt, juice and cayenne pepper, till very smooth. Serve and change the seasonings. Decorate with some new herbs.

If you prepare Dr. Sebi's Cleansing Green Soup, you are requested to please take a photo and share with the world on Sebi 's Official page of Facebook. We love if you share your experience with us.

4.2. Bell Pepper and Roasted Tomato Soup

Serving: 2

Total Time: 50 Minutes

Ingredients:

- Ripe Roma tomatoes 4

- red bell peppers 3

- fresh sprigs thyme 3

- Vegetable broth homemade 1/4 cup (make it with approved vegetables only)

- sea salt 100% pure according to your taste and some sesame oil

Directions:

Preheat your oven at 375 degrees F. Chop the peppers in quarter then cut the cores. Slice the tomatoes and put the bell peppers onto rimmed baking dish. Drizzle completely with the sesame oil and dust with sea salt. Spread the thyme all over the vegetables. Roast for about 35-40 minutes in a heated oven. Move everything into a blender or a food processor. Include the heated broth and the puree till it looks smooth, add more broth if required to obtain the perfect consistency.

Apply salt as per your taste. Pour in the bowls and serve.

4.3. Chickpea Soup

Serving: 4

Total Time: 30 minutes

Ingredients:

- Chickpeas 2 cups

- Zucchini 1 small size

- Bell pepper1

- Small onion1

- Water as required

- Seasoning with own choice

Directions:

Place all things in a pot and simmer over medium heat till vegetables are aldente. As soon as the soup gets ready and vegetables are cooked, take a multi-purpose blender and then blend them well. That's the best way to enjoy that. This is going to produce a soup for a couple of days.

4.4. Kale Soup

Serving: 2

Total Time: 30 minutes

Ingredients:

- onion chopped 1 medium size

- vegetable broth 5 cups

- chayote, diced 1 medium size

- squash, diced 2 cups

- kale 3 cups, rinsed, removed stems and fine chopped

- dried thyme 2 tbs

- dried sage two tbs

- pepper and salt as per taste

Directions:

Chop the onions and let them stay for 5 minutes. Warm one tabs of the broth in a medium pot. Saute the onion in the broth on medium heat, constantly stirring for 5 minutes. Add the broth and the chayote and bring to a boil. After heating, decrease the heat and proceed to cook for another

five min. Add squash and simmer for around 15 min until soft. Add kale and remaining ingredients and simmer for another 5 mins. You want to cook longer for more taste and richness, then you may have to add a little more broth.

4.5. Alkaline Electric Soup

Serving:4

Total Time: 1.5 Hour

Ingredients:

- Approved Pasta/ Kamut Pasta 1-2 cups

- Quinoa Optional, 1/2 cup

- (cooked) Garbanzo Beans* 1/2 lb.

- Mushrooms, chopped 2 cups

- chopped Zucchini Squash 1

- chopped, Butternut Squash, 2 cups

- Green Peppers chopped, 1/2 cup

- Red Peppers chopped 1/2 cup

- chopped Red Onion small size, 1

- diced Roma Tomatoes, 2

- Spring Water 1/2 Gallon (adjust as required)

- Dill 1 tbs

- Red Cayenne Pepper 1 tbs

- Grapeseed Oil 1 tbs

- Oregano 1 tbs

- Basil 1 tbs

- Sea Salt 1 tbs

Directions:

Soak garbanzo beans in water overnight and boil them just before adding them to the Native Stew.

Pour spring water into a big pot and set the flame on medium heat.

Chop off all the herbs. Add the ingredients with seasonings to the pot and boil for around 1 hour. Stir the mixture every 15 minutes. Freeze the remaining stew for another day!

4.6. Greens Soup

Serving: 2

Total Time: 1 Hour

Ingredients:

- leafy greens 2 cups

- zucchini 1 small

- bell pepper 1

- onion 1 small

- Water as required

- Seasoning as per choice

Directions:

Put all ingredients in a pot and then cook over medium heat til the vegetables get semi-hard. Switch off the burner, let it cool and mix well together.

4.7. Ginger Soup / Electric Alkaline Soursop

Serving: 6-8

Total Time: 1.5 Hours

Ingredients:

- Soursop Leaves 4-6

- spring water 12-16 cups (1 gallon=16 cups)

- chopped kale 2 cups

- One whole cubed chayote squash, or 2 cups

- zucchini cubed 1 cup

- cubed summer squash 1 cup

- diced onions 1 cup

- green peppers diced 1 cup

- red peppers diced 1 cup

- Quinoa 1 cup (wild rice only approved / pasta /grain)

- onion powder 3 tbs

- sea salt four tbs

- basil 1 tbs

- oregano 1 tbs

- minced fresh ginger, one tbs

- cayenne (optional) 1/4 teaspoon

Directions:

Rinse the soursop leaves and rip them in half, then put them in a big pot with four cups of spring water. Boil the leaves for 15-20 minutes with the pot cover. Drop the leaves of the soup. Add rest of the ingredients. Add 8 cups of spring water. (for making quinoa You may add more water if you use grains/rice that consume more water) Stir in the spices, cover the lid and simmer on medium heat for 30 to 45 minutes. (More time could be required if you do not use quinoa).

4.8. Chayote Mushroom Soup (Stew)

Serving: 6-8

Total Time: 40 min

Ingredients:

- Spring Water 6 cups

- Sliced Mushrooms, 3 cups

- Cubed Chayote Squash, 2 cups

- Some Chickpea Flour or the Garbanzo Bean flour 1 & half cups

- diced Onions 1 cup

- Vegetable Broth* or Aquafaba 1 cup

- Hemp Milk 1 cup

- Grapeseed Oil 1-2 tbps.

- Onion Powder 1 tbps.

- Sea Salt 2 tsp.

- Basil 2 tsp

- Red Pepper Crushed1 tsp

- Whisk or Blender

Directions:

* Water is the alternative if you don't have any of them peel the skin of chayote squash, and break it into cubes. Apply the grapeseed oil to the broad pot and sauté the mushrooms and onions for about 3-5 minutes over medium-high heat. Pour 4 cups of spring water, milk, chayote, aquafaba and seasonings into a pot and stir. Then cover with lid on medium heat. Now Add garbanzo-bean flour. After that add the leftover 2 cups of water into the blender and swirl for 20 sec. Or until no chunks are visible. You may even whisk the two ingredients together in cup. Add the mixture to the pot again and boil over low heat about 30 min. stir periodically. Enjoy the hot Alkaline Electric soup of Chayote-Mushroom!

4.9. Mushroom Soup

Serving: 6

Total Time: 45 minutes

Ingredients:

Grapeseed Oil 2 tbsp.

Sliced Mushrooms, 3 cups

Cayenne Powder 1 tsp.

Garbanzo Beans Flour 1 ½ cup

Basil, torn 2 tsp.

Mashed Onion 1 cup,

Pure Sea Salt 2 tsp.

Chayote Squash 2 cups, (peeled & cubed)

Onion Powder 1 tbsp.

Hempseed Milk 1 cup

Cayenne Pepper 1 tsp.

Aquafaba 1 cup

Directions:

Start with a spoonful of oil in a big pot and cook over low heat. When the oil has become mildly sweet, mix onion and the mushrooms. Cook them for about 5 minutes or till clear and soft. Next, a spoon full of hemp seed oil, aquafaba, and 4 cups of spring. Add water to the pot. Then mix the cubes of the squash with seasonings. Get the mixture to boil. In the meanwhile, combine the flour of garbanzo bean with the leftover flour. Add Spring water into the blender for about 1 to 2 minutes or till smooth. And no lumps. Finally, add the flour mixture into the pot and put it all for a good mix. Cook the solution for 30 min. or until the mixture gets thicked.

4.10. Gazpacho Soup

Serving: 2

Total Time: 5 minutes

Ingredients:

- Spring Water 2 cups

- Basil 2 Leaves

- Ripe Avocado 1

- Juice of 1 Lime

- peeled Cucumber without seeds 1

- Pure Sea Salt ¼ tsp.

Directions:

To start, put all ingredients, except sea salt, in a cup. In the oven. Then put all ingredients into a high-speed blender for blending about 1-2 minutes, or before you have a smooth broth with a little bit of Its chunk. Next, put the soup into a tub and hold it in the refrigerator.

4.11. Chayote Mushroom Soup

Serving: 10

Total Time: 10 minutes

Ingredients:

- Hemp Milk, 1 cup

- Crushed Red Pepper, 1 tsp.

- Onion Powder, 1 tbsp.

- Sliced Mushroom, 3 cups

- Diced Onion, 1 cup

- Chayote Squash 2 cups, cubed

- Sea Salt 2 tsp.

- Basil 2 tsp.

- Grapeseed Oil 2 tbsp.

- Vegetable Broth 1 cup

- Garbanzo Flour 1 ½ cup

- Spring Water 6 cups

Directions:

Firstly, over medium-high fire, put a large saucepan. Add a spoon of the once it gets warmed, stir in the oil and add Champignons and onions. Then add the milk, other seasonings, 4 cups of chayote with 4 cups of chayote, add spring water in it, and then include vegetable broth then cover with lid. Next, add garbanzo flour, pass the mixture into a blender. Now, combine the mixture for about 15-20 sec. or until the mixture is fully mixed. There shouldn't be any lumps. Transfer mixture into the pan until combined and simmer it for 30 minutes. Serve hot and enjoy.

Chapter 5. Dr. Sebi Salads

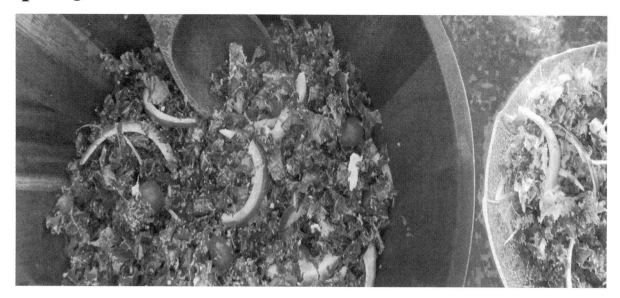

5.1. Romaine Lettuce Salad (Grilled)

Serving: 1

Total time: 30 mins.

Ingredients:

- Romaine lettuce 4 small heads, washed

- Key lime juice 1 tbsp.

- Red onion 1 tbsp., cut into fine pieces

- Onion powder as per taste

- Sea salt as per taste

- Fresh basil 1 tbsp., cut into fine pieces

- Cayenne pepper as per taste

- Agave syrup 1 tbsp.

- Olive oil 4 tbsp.

Directions:

Place the cut side of the lettuce half in a wide nonstick tray. Don't apply some oil to it. Turn over the lettuce to check its hue. Made sure that the lettuce is golden brown on both ends. Turn off the heat, remove the pan, and let the lettuce cool down on a large plate. In a tiny mixing cup, add the red onion with the olive oil, the key lime juice, the agave syrup and the new basil. Now as per taste, add the salt and pepper. Whisk to mix it well. Take a serving dish, put the grilled lettuce into this dish. Now drizzle it with the dressing and enjoy it.

Did you like this dish? Next, try our Watercress Citrus Salad and the Alkaline-Electric Salad. Let's see which one will be your favorite.

5.2. Strawberry Salad with Dandelion

Serving: 4

Total time: 50 mins.

Ingredients:

- Grape-seed oil 2 tbsp.

- Strawberries 10, must be ripe one, chopped

- Red onion one medium, chopped

- Dandelion greens 4 cups

- Key lime juice 2 tbsp.

- Sea salt as per taste

Directions:

Take a nonstick pan (of 12-inch), put grapeseed oil in it and heat it over medium flame. Now add sea salt (1 pinch) and the sliced onions in the pan. Cook, stirring regularly until the onions are smooth, softly golden and decreased to about one-third of the raw amount.

In a little cup, add one teaspoon of the key lime juice in the strawberry slices. Clean the dandelion greens and break them into bite-sized bits if you prefer. Once the onions are almost done, pour the rest of the key lime juice into the pan, then cook for a few minutes till the onions are browned. Remove the ointment from heat. In the salad cup, mix the onions, greens and strawberries along with all of the juices. Sprinkle the sea salt and enjoy.

5.3. Avocado Basil Pasta Salad

Serving: 6

Total time: 15 mins.

Ingredients:

- Avocado 1, sliced

- Fresh basil 1 cup, sliced

- Cherry tomatoes 1-pint, cut into two halves

- Key lime juice 1 tbsp.

- Agave syrup 1 tsp.

- Olive oil 1/4 cup

- Spelt-pasta 4 cups, cooked or any other pasta, accepted by Dr. Sebi's book "Cell-Food Nutritional Guide."

Directions:

In a wide tub, put the cooked pasta. Add the tomatoes, basil and avocado and stir until the components have been completely combined. In a tiny cup, blend well together with the oil, the agave syrup, the lime juice, and the sea salt. Mix with the pasta and blend to combine.

5.4. Watercress Citrus Salad (Detox Salad)

Serving: 6

Total time: 10 mins.

Ingredients:

- An avocado must be ripe

- Watercress 4 cups

- Seville orange 1, skinned and sliced

- Red onion 2, cut into very thin pieces

- Agave syrup 2 tsp.

- Key lime juice 2 tsp.

- Olive oil 2 tsp.

- Salt 1/8 tsp.

- Cayenne pepper is optional as per your taste.

Directions:

Arrange the watercress, the avocado, the onion and the orange on two dishes. Mix well the lime juice, the agave syrup, olive oil, salt and the cayenne pepper in a shallow dish. Prepare the serving bowl by placing a spoon as dressing over salad as it's about to eat. Enjoy!

5.5 Headache Averting Salad

Serving: 3

Total time: 7 mins.

Ingredients:

- Seeded cucumber 1/2

- Watercress 2 cups

- Olive oil 2 tbsp.

- Key lime juice 1 tbsp.

- Cayenne pepper as per taste

- Sea salt as per taste

Directions:

Mix well the olive oil with the key lime. Arrange the watercress and the cucumber. Add the seasoning and, for taste, spray with the salt and the pepper. Enjoy the delicious salad.

5.6. Cherry Tomato Salad

Serving: 5

Total time: 10 mins.

Ingredients:

- Cherry tomatoes 4 cups

- Red onion 1/4 cup, sliced

- Herbs like dill, sweet basil,

- Olive oil, 1/4 cup

- The Key lime juice 1 1/2 tbsp.

- Date sugar 1/4 teaspoon

- Salt as per taste

- Cayenne pepper as required

Directions:

Preparing the cherry tomato salad begins with putting the tomatoes into a wide bowl and then adding the red onion and the herbs. Now, let's bring on the dressing! Take a tiny cup, mix together the olive oil, along with the date syrup, the lime juice, the sea salt and the cayenne pepper according to taste.

Add the dressing into the mixture of tomatoes and swirl gently to cover uniformly. Serve, and have fun! Have you liked this recipe? Follow Dr. Sebi's recipes and find out more ideas and information about cooking!

5.7. Dr. Sebi's special Mango Salad

Serving: 4

Total time: 45 mins.

Ingredients:

- Mangoes 2

- Red onion 1/4

- Cherry tomatoes 1/4 cup

- Cucumber 1/2, having seeds

- Bell pepper ½, green

- Key lime 1

- Sea salt according to taste

- Cayenne pepper according to taste

Directions:

Preparing Mango Salad begins with cutting the mangoes, chopping the red onion, and slicing the cherry tomatoes. Slice thinly the seeded cucumber as well as the bell pepper. In a little tub, add all the ingredients and mix. Take the lime and spill over the salad.

Sprinkle with salt and cayenne pepper and leave for marinating in the refrigerator for about 20 minutes before feeding. Enjoy it as your salad, a salsa or even a dip, that's your call!

5.8. Cucumber Salad (Asian Style)

Serving: 1

Total time: 5 mins.

Ingredients:

- Key lime juice three tbs.

- Sesame oil 1 tbs.

- Date sugar 1/2 tsp.

- Sea salt 1/4 tsp.

- Ginger 1 tbs., in grated form

- Sesame seeds 1 tbs.

- Seaweed 1 tbs., in powdered granulated form

Direction:

To cook the Asian Cucumber Salad, simply pour it all together and enjoy it!

5.9. Basic Electric Chickpea or Bengal Gram Salad ("Tuna" Salad)

Serving: 2-4

Total Time: 1 hour 15 mins.

Ingredients

- Chickpeas 2 cups, properly cooked

- Basic Electric Hemp Seed Mayo 2/3 cup

- Red Onions 1/4 cup, chopped

- Green Peppers 1/8 cup, cubed

- Dulse Granules 1 tbsp. or Nori Sheet 1/2

- Onion Powder 2 tsp.

- Dill 1 tsp.

- Sea Salt 1/4 tsp.

- Masher

Dimensions:

Take chickpeas and add into the bowl and grind until the optimal texture has been achieved. If a sheet of Nori is used, split into tiny pieces and mix with the chickpeas. Mix the remaining

ingredients to the bowl and blend well. Keep it in refrigerator to cool for about 30 − 60 minutes before eating. Enjoy the Alkaline Electric Chickpea "Tuna" Salad!

5.10. Electric Pasta Salad (Alkaline)

Serving: 5-7

Total Time: 30 mins.

Ingredients

- Spelt Pasta/Basic Homemade Pasta 4 cups, cooked

- Bell Peppers 1 cup, either Red, Yellow or Green, cubed

- Zucchini/Summer Squash 1 cup, chopped

- Onions 1/2 cup, chopped

- Cherry Tomatoes 1/2 cup, cut them in two halves

- Black Olives 1/4 cup

- Alkaline "Garlic" Sauce 3/4 to 1 cup

Directions

Toss all the ingredients in a wide bowl once well combined and enjoy the Electric Pasta Salad (alkaline).

5.11. Quinoa Zucchini Salad

Serving: 12-14 slices

Total time: 50 mins.

Ingredients:

- Oregano 1 tsp.

- Spring Onion 2, finely sliced

- Olive Oil 3 tbsp.

- Zucchini 2, must be large & chopped

- Grapeseed Oil 2 tbsp.

- Key Lime Juice 1

- Chickpeas 15 oz. can

- Onion Powder 1 tsp.

- Quinoa 5 cup, properly cooked

Directions

First of all, take a tablespoon of oil into a large frying pan over medium flame. After this, now mix it in the slices of zucchini and simmer for three to four minutes or before tendering. Next is spooning in oregano and pour the residual oil into the pan.

In the final step, add cooked zucchini with the rest of the ingredients to a large bowl. Now toss well. It's ready to enjoy.

5.12. Chickpeas (Bengali Gram) Salad

Serving: 3

Total times: 10 mins.

Ingredients:

- Chickpeas (Bengali gram) 1 ½ cups, drained & washed

- Red Onion ½ cup, cubed

- Cilantro ¼ cup, fresh one & well chopped

- Avocado 1 cup

- Sea Salt as per taste

Directions

First, put the chickpeas (Bengali gram) in a wide bowl then mash it with the masher. After doing this mash, the avocado now and then mixes it properly. In this mixture, add lemon juice and blend properly. Then whisk with the lime juice, blend and mix with the cilantro. Stir it again. Then, a spoon of salt. Whisk it again.

Serve and enjoy yourself.

5.13. Cucumber Mushroom Salad

Serving: 2.

Total time: 15 mins.

Ingredients:

- Olive Oil 1 tsp.

- Mushrooms 5, cut into two halves

- Key Lime Juice ½ of 1

- Olives 10

- Cherry Tomatoes 6, cut into two halves

- Sea Salt, as desired

- Lettuce leaves 6, rinsed

- Cucumber ½ of 1, sliced

Directions

Put the lettuce leaves, onions, mushrooms, olives, and cucumber in a wide mixing bowl to create this simple, balanced salad. After this, spill a spoon of olive oil along with the key lime juice on the salad. Toss it well. In the last, pour the sea salt on it. Toss the mixture well. Now enjoy yourself.

5.14. Fruit Salad (Citrus)

Serving: 4

Total time: 50 mins.

Ingredients:

- Grapes 8 oz., seeded one

- Key Lime 1, should be quartered

- Medjool Dates 8, cut into two halves

- Kiwi 2, sliced

- Seville Oranges 4, skinned & sliced

Directions:

First, position all the ingredients required to produce the salad, excluding lime, in a wide mixing bowl. After this, squeeze the lime and pour it all over the salad, then toss properly. Serve, enjoy and love yourself.

5.15. Mashed Squash Salad

Serving: 6

Total time: 10 mins.

Ingredients:

- Allspice 1 tsp.

- Blue Agave ¼ cup, natural

- Squash 2, skinned & cubed

- Sea Salt 1/8 tsp.

- Date Sugar ¼ cup

- Hemp Milk ¼ cup

Directions

To start with, put the squash chunks and the water in a saucepan over medium flame. Boil the mixture and simmer for twenty minutes or when the squash is soft. When soft, clear the water then mash the squash. After this, add a spoon of date sugar, organic milk, allspice, sea salt and agave. Mix it well. Serve yourself and love it.

5.16. Watercress Salad

Serving: 2

Total time: 15 mins.

Ingredients:

- 1/8 tsp. Pure Sea Salt

- 4 cups Watercress, torn

- 2 tbsp. Olive Oil

- 1 Avocado, pitted, halved and sliced

- 2 tsp. Agave Syrup

- Cayenne Powder, as needed

- 2 Red Onions, sliced thinly

- 1 Seville Orange, peeled & cubed

- 2 tbsp. Key Lime Juice

Directions

First, take a mixing bowl, add orange, avocado, onion, and watercress. Now take another mixing bowl and add olive oil, the cayenne powder, key lime juice, agave syrup and the sea salt. Mix them well. Now, pour the olive oil dressing on the salad then toss it well. Serve the nutritious salad, enjoy and love it thoroughly.

Chapter 6: Dr. Sebi's Main Courses

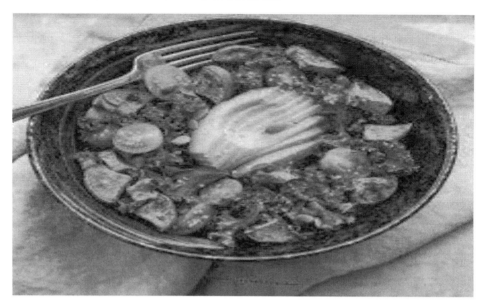

6.1. Mushrooms with Wild Rice

Serving: 3

Total Time: 8 minutes

Ingredients:

- Finely chopped mushrooms, 1 cup

- Olive Oil 1 tsp.

- Sea Salt 1 tsp.

- Wild Rice, cooked 1 cup

- Kale ½ cup

Directions:

Start cooking the kale in medium-sized skillet along with a little oil. Over medium flame. Cook the ingredients for 2-3 minutes or till mildly wilted. Keep it aside on a tray. Reserve the oil therein. Then, mix in the pan with the mushrooms and simmer for 3-5 minutes. Transfer mushrooms to plate until they are browned. Next, season with salt and pepper on mushroom. Serve it with, wild rice and kale.

6.2. Quinoa Rice

Serving: 2

Total Time: 50 minutes

Ingredients:

- Diced Onion, ¼ of 1.

- Cooked Quinoa 1 cup.

- Cubed Bell Pepper, ½ of 1.

- Grape-seed Oil ½ tbsp.

- Cubed Zucchini ½ cup.

- 100% Pure Sea-Salt ½ tsp.

- Sliced Mushroom, ½ cup.

- Cayenne Pepper as required or ¼ tsp.

Directions:

Add a spoon of oil in a low heated medium-sized pan to make this wonderful rice dish. Once the oil is warmed, mix the onion in it and cook it for 4 minutes. Or till slightly browned. Then, add a spoon of onions, zucchini and bell peppers, mix it with the onion and bell peppers. Keep cooking for an extra 4 minutes or till the vegetables are soft.

Now, stir in the saucepan the cooked quinoa then blend well until it's done. When everything is mixed together, and the rice gets soft, stop cooking it. Finally, place them in a bowl and serve.

6.3. Amaranth with Pears

Serving: 4

Total Time: 15 minutes

Ingredients:

- Chopped Walnuts & Currants ½ cup

- Amaranth 1 cup

- Salt 1 Pinch

- Spring Water 3 cups

- Agave Syrup 1 tbsp.

- Pear half of 1

- Coconut Oil 1 tbsp.

Directions:

In a pan, add some water. Boil the water, then mix amaranth and cook until it starts to boil. Now let it boil for 9-12 minutes or till it is done. Stir frequently. When the mixture continues to thicken, Remove the pan from the burner for a creamy consistency. Next, add the remaining ingredients into another saucepan. Offer it a gentle stir. Cook for 2-3 minutes over medium heat. Ultimately, add the blend into cooked amaranth; after that, mix everything properly.

6.4. Garbanzo Bean Burger

Serving: 4

Total Time: 40 minutes

Ingredients:

- Cayenne Pepper ½ tsp.

- Garbanzo Flour 1 cup

- Sea Salt 100% Pure 2 tsp.

- Diced Kale, ½ cup

- Cayenne Powder ½ tsp.

- diced Plum Tomato, 1

- Dill 1 tsp.

- diced Green Peppers ½ cup,

- Oregano 2 tsp.

- Diced Onion, ½ cup

- Spring Water ½ cup

- Basil 2 tsp.

- Grape-seed Oil 2 tbsp.

- Onion Powder 2 tsp.

- For the burger:

- 8 Flatbreads

- Sauce1 cup

- Tomatoes Plum, sliced 2

- sliced Red Onion, 1

Directions:

In a wide mixing cup, blend all the spices along with vegetables and add the garbanzo flour. Steadily pour spring water. Combine it all until you get a dough. Tip: Apply more flour if you need to harden the dough. Create the cutlets from this dough now. Start heating oil over medium heat in a medium-sized pan. Once the oil gets hot, reduce the heat to mild. Cook the cutlets for about 4 minutes, or until they are golden brown.

Take flatbread and place the burger inside along with Tomato, pepper, and gravy. Serve and enjoy the recipe.

6.5. Chickpea French Fries

Serving: 8

Total Time: 1 hour and 45 minutes

Ingredients:

- Sea Salt, 1 tsp.

- Minced, ½ cup Onion

- Chickpea Flour, 2 cups

- Cayenne, 1 tsp.

- Oregano, 1 tbsp.

- Green Bell Peppers ½ cup, diced

- Grapeseed Oil, 2 tbsp.

- Spring Water, 4 cups

- Onion Powder, 1 tbsp.

Directions:

You have to boil water in a wide area to create this lip-smacking dish. Start with medium heat, and gradually reduce and mix in the flour of the chickpea. The onions, spices, and bell pepper are next to it. Cook the mixture of chickpeas for 10 mins. Or until it is thickened while stirs it after sometimes. Now, spill the mixture over a baking sheet lined with parchment paper. Greased with tar. Cover mixture with spatula thinly and hold the leftover parchment on top. Next, put the sheet for about 20 mins in the freezer.

Cut in any manner as desired when time is finished. Preheat oven to 400 ° F or 200 ° C; after that, take one more baking sheet lined with parchment paper, greased with oil, and the bits are kept in it. For 20 minutes, roast them. Flip them over. Keep cooking for ten more minutes, or before they are brown or golden. Serve them hot.

6.6. Zucchini Pasta

Serving: 2

Total Time: 25 minutes

Ingredients:

- large & Spiralized, Zucchini 4

- Sea Salt, ¼ tsp.

- Avocadoes Medium-sized, 2.

- Grape-seed Oil, 2 tbsp.

- Cherry Tomatoes, 1 cup.

- Fresh Basil ¼ cup.

Directions:

Start with a spiralizer to spiral the zucchini, create thin strips with Peeler's help for herbs. After that, add a spoon of oil on medium heat, use a large skillet. Mix in zoodles and cook for 4-5 minutes or till the zoodles are ready fried and tender. Withdraw from the heat. Shift to a wide serving dish. Add cherry tomatoes, salt avocados, basil, and mix everything well. Mix everything and serve.

6.7. Kale with Pepper

Serving: 4

Total Time: 25 minutes

Ingredients:

- Diced, Red Pepper 1 tbs

- Kale 1 bunch, (washed & pat dried)

- Grape Seed Oil, 1 tsp.

- Diced Onion ¼ cup,

- Sea Salt, ¼ tsp.

- Crushed Chili 1 tsp,

Directions:

Begin by taking dried kale, fold each kale in half. Slice and stem off. Tear the leaves into smaller pieces. Add some oil into a pan and heat over high flame. Mix onion, pepper and iodine. Cook for three minutes. Reduce heat to a low. Now, add kale and cook for 5 minutes. Stir in crushed red pepper and offer a nice swirl to all. Cook until soft or about 3 minutes. Remove from the heat and serve.

6.8. Baked Nuts

Serving:4

Total Time:20 minutes

Ingredients:

- Hemp Seeds, ½ cup

- Walnuts 1 cup; Olive Oil 1 tsp

- Brazil Nuts 1 cup; Sesame Seeds 1 tsp

Directions:

Start by preheating the oven to 350 F. Next, in a mixing cup, blend both the nuts and the hemp-seeds until mixed. Up, right. And sesame seeds on top. Finally, bake for between 18 to 20 mins. Let it to cool and serve.

6.9. Energy Balls

Serving: 1

Total Time: 20 minutes

Ingredients:

- Salt ¼ tsp.

- Brazil Nuts ¾ cup; Coconut Oil 2 tbsp.

- Walnuts ¾ cup; Dried Fruits ¼ cup

- Sesame Seeds ½ cup; Hemp Hearts ½ cup, Figs ½ cup, dried

Directions:

Start by putting the seeds (sesame), figs, salt in the food processor and Mix them all for 2-3 minutes or till a sticky blend is produced. Shift to a tub.

Put Brazil nuts and walnuts in the processor and then mix till they convert into a texture yet crumbly. Add the walnut blend to the mixture with sesame seeds.

Merge and mix with spoon in the fruits or hemp hearts until mixed. Mix and Combine the mixture with coconut. Finally, create rolls from the blend and store them all in air-tight jar.

6.10. Baked Kale Chips

Serving: 4

Total Time: 20 minutes.

Ingredients:

- Kale 1 lb, washed & patted dry

- Sea Salt Pure, as needed

- Grapeseed Oil, 1 tbsp.

- as needed, Cayenne Pepper

Directions:

Preheat your oven to 350 degrees F. Tear off leaves from kale and stem; after that place grapeseed oil, kale leaves, cayenne pepper and sea salt in the mixture. Add everything to a mixing bowl. Soak the kale leaves with seasoning and then put them for baking on the Parchment-paper-lined sheet. Next, cook for eight minutes or till they get crispy.

6.11. Macaroni & Cheese

Serving: 8-10

Total Time: 15 minutes

Ingredients:

- Hemp Milk, 1 cup

- Kamut Pasta, 12 oz.

- Pure Sea Salt, 1 tsp.

- All Spice, ½ tsp.

- Flour of Garbanzo Bean, ¼ cup.

- Brazil Nuts ½ lb, raw & soaked

- ½ Juice of 1 Lime

- Spring Water, 1 cup

- Onion Powder, 2 tsp.

- Grape-seed Oil, 2 tsp.

Directions:

Cook the pasta to render this balanced food by following Instructions as given on the packet. Pre-heat your oven to 350 ° F. Then, using a high-speed blender, put all the ingredients required to produce the dressing. Blend the mixture for 2 minutes or before it becomes all smooth. Now, over medium-high flame, heat oil in a broad skillet. Mix the pasta and simmer for 1 minute until the oil becomes hot.

Next, add the sauce over the skillet and give it all a gentle swirl. Lastly, cook pasta for about 30 minutes or till it's fully cooked.

6.12. Sautéed Greens

Serving: 8-10

Total Time: 15 minutes

Ingredients:

- Turnip Green, three bunches

- Pure Sea Salt, 3 tbsp.

- Onions 2 cups, chopped

- Cayenne Pepper, 1 tsp.

- Olive Oil, 1 tbsp.

Directions:

To begin, in a medium skillet, Saute onion over medium heat. After frying, add greens and roast for 18-20 minutes. Finally, season the mixture with cayenne pepper and salt.

6.13. Veggie Quinoa

Serving: 6-8

Total Time: 15 minutes

Ingredients:

- Basil, 1 tsp.

- Quinoa cooked 4 cups.

- Oregano 1 tsp.

- Zucchini chopped 1 cup.

- Pure Sea Salt 2 tsp.

- Red Bell Pepper ¼ cup, chopped

- Onion ½ cup, diced

- Green Bell Pepper¼ cup, chopped

- Cayenne Pepper ½ tsp.

- Yellow Bell Pepper ¼ cup, chopped

- Tomato 1 Plum, chopped

- Spring Water ½ cup

- Onion Powder 1 tbsp.

- Grape-seed Oil 2 tbsp.

Directions:

Begin by adding oil in a wide pan over medium heat. Then stir vegetables and season with the mixture and cook it for five minutes or before tender. Now, dump in the water together with the quinoa. Give it a nice swirl and finish cooking for two more minutes. Serve it.

6.14. Teff Porridge

Serving: 2

Total Time: 20 minutes

Ingredients:

- Spring Water, 2 cups

- Teff Grain 5 cups

- Sea Salt as required

- Agave Syrup 2 tbsp.

Directions:

First, boil the water into a pot on medium-high heat, then, as soon as it begins, Boil, whisk in the teff, then add the salt. Cover pot with the lid and lower the heat. Now, boil it for 10-15 minutes or till cooked. Serve with the seasoning of agave syrup and blueberries and serve.

6.15. Apple Quinoa Porridge

Serving:4

Total Time: 20 minutes

Ingredients:

- Key Lime ½ of 1

- Quinoa 5 cup; Apple 1 grated

- Coconut Oil 1 tbsp; Ginger 1-inch

Directions:

Begin with cooking the quinoa using the given instructions set on the envelope. Add the apple for five minutes until cooked. Now, simmer for half a minute and then add in the zest of lemon. The juice of the lemon to it. Next, stir the coconut oil, and mix well. Finally, scatter the mixture in the serving bowls. Garnish with the ginger.

6.16. Alkaline Electric Zucchini Bacon

Serving: 2-4

Total Time: 2 hours

Ingredients:

- Zucchini 2-3

- Date Sugar 1/4 cup

- Spring Water 1/4 cup

- Agave 2 tbsp.

- Sea Salt Smoked 1 tbsp.

- Onion Powder 1 tbsp.

- Liquid Smoke 1 tsp.

- Cayenne Powder 1/2 tsp.

- Ginger Powder 1/2 tsp.

- Mandoline / Potato Peeler

- Paper Parchment

- Grapeseed Oil

Directions:

Add all the ingredients into the saucepan and steam over low heat, and wait till they dissolved. Chop the zucchini and use the potato peeler to create the strips. In a wide bowl, mix the zucchini with the saucepan's ingredients and marinate for 30 to 60 minutes. There is no need for more water since it will come from zucchini. Use parchment paper on to the baking sheet and cover slightly with grape-seed oil. Cover the sheet with marinated strips, and bake at 400 ° F for ten minutes. Flip zucchini strips, cook 3-4 minutes, then leave to cool. If you like any of the strips to be crispy, roast for few more minutes or fry in a finely oiled pan for 30 sec. Enjoy the Alkaline-Electric-Bacon of Zucchini.

6.17. Vegetable Omelet

Serving: 1

Total Time: 25 minutes

Ingredients:

- Oregano ¼ tsp.

- Flour (Garbanzo Beans) ¼ cup

- Chopped Mushrooms ¼ cup

- Chopped Roma Tomato, ¼ cup

- Diced Green Pepper, ¼ cup

- Chopped Onion ¼ cup,

- Sea Salt 100% Pure ¼ tsp.

- Grapeseed Oil 1 tbsp.

- Onion Powder ¼ tsp

- Spring Water 1/3 cup

- Basil, sweet ¼ tsp.

- Cayenne Powder ¼ tsp.

Directions:

Start by putting garbanzo bean flour, include water and add seasoning in a wide mixing bowl. Whisk the combination properly, so it is properly blended. Heat oil in a large skillet on medium-high heat. When the oil is warmed, mix in a spoonful of all vegetables and the tomatoes. Sautee it for 2-3 minutes or before it becomes slightly tender.

Now add the flour mixture over it and blend it properly. Cook the mixture for 4 minutes, then turn mixture side by side. Using a spatula, remove the omelet's sides and turn it gently to the elevated position such that all parts of the omelet can be lifted. Only get fried. Serve them warm, please.

6.18. Macaroni & Cheese

Serving: 10

Total Time: 45 minutes

Ingredients:

- Grapeseed Oil 2 tsp.

- Alkaline Pasta 12 oz.

- Juice 1 of ½ Key Lime

- Onion Powder 2 tsp.

- Garbanzo Flour ¼ cup

- Sea Salt 1 tsp.

- Spring Water 1 cup

- Raw Brazil Nuts 1 cup, overnight soaked

- Hempseed Milk 1 cup

- Achiote, grounded ½ tsp.

Directions:

Cook the pasta first according to the directions on the packet. Then, heat the oven to 350 F. Place the cooked pasta and drizzle oil over it into a baking dish. In a high-speed mixer, put all remaining ingredients and mix until the sauce gets creamy for 2 min or until ticked. Stir the cooked pasta with the sauce and chop it properly. Bake pasta for 20-30 minutes.

6.19. Mango Papaya Seed Dressing

Serving: 2

Total time: 3 mins.

- Ingredients

- Chopped Mango, 1 cup

- Grapeseed Oil 1/4 cup

- Lime Juice 2 tbsp.

- Ground Papaya Seed 1 tsp.

- Agave 1 tsp.

- Basil 1 tsp.

- Onion Powder 1 tsp.

- Sea Salt 1/4 tsp.

Directions:

Blend the ingredients inside blender and blend them for about a minute, it is now ready to serve.

6.20. Cucumber Dill Dressing

Serving: 2

Total time: 3 mins.

Ingredients:

- Chopped Plum Tomatoes, 2

- Sesame Seeds2 tbsp.

- Minced Onion, 1 tbsp.

- Agave 1 tbsp.

- Lime Juice 1 tbsp.

- Minced Ginger, 1 tsp.

Directions:

Start by blending all the ingredients in a blender and blend them for about 1&half minute, it is now ready to serve.

6.21 Alkaline Electric Mushroom & Onion Gravy

Serving: 3

Total time: 13 mins.

Ingredients:

- Spring Water 2-3 cups
- Mushrooms 1/2 cup
- Onions 1/2 Cup
- Garbanzo bean flour 3 tbs.
- Grapeseed Oil 2 tbs.
- Sea Salt 1 tsp.
- Onion Powder 1 tsp.
- Oregano 1/2 tsp.
- Thyme 1/2 tsp.
- Cayenne 1/4 tsp.

Directions:

Stir in skillet with grapeseed oil for about 2 minutes and Saute mushrooms & onions with all spices and seasonings, bar cayenne.

Add about 2 cups spring water. Then add cayenne powder and cook for five minutes. Mix it all up and get it to a boil. Proceed to cook to simmer, if necessary you can add remaining water. Enjoy your Alkaline Mushroom & Onion Gravy or your favorite meal with Kamut.

6.22 Alkaline Electric Vegan "Ribs"

Serving: 3

Total time: 8 Hours.

Ingredients:

- Mushrooms Portobello 2

- Alkaline Barbecue Sauce 1/2 cup

- Spring Water 1/4 cup

- Sea Salt 1 tsp.

- Onion powder 1 tsp.

- Cayenne 1/2 tsp.

- Grapeseed oil 2 tbs

Directions:

Scrape off gills for each mushroom cap 's underside in order to prevent an earthy flavor and split mushrooms roughly 1/2 inch apart. dd mushrooms then add spices, water and much barbecue sauce in a wide tub. Cover with cap, shake and store for around 6-8 hours in the refrigerator. After every 2 hours, flip bottle. Take a skewer and force 3 mushrooms chop around the middle, add another skewer, and fill in another 2-3 bits. If slices split, you may cook them as snacks.

rush the olive oil over medium heat, and start cook the ribs for 12-15 minutes, tossing every 3 minutes. you may be rush more sauce barbecue, if a few flips are needed. Serve hot and enjoy.

Chapter 7: Dr. Sebi's Dessert

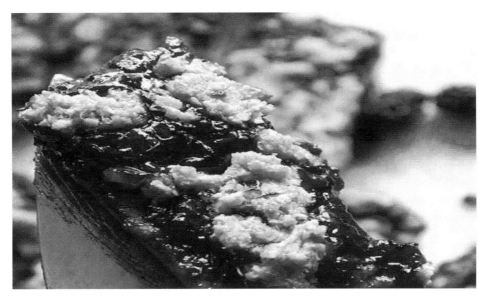

7.1 Berry Brownie Pizza (No-Bake)

Serving: 8-10

Total time: 25 mins.

Ingredients

- Walnuts or pecans 2.5 cups, raw form

- Pitted dates 2.5 cups

- Cacao powder ½ cup

- Salt, a large pinch

- Coffee or water 1–2 tbsp., brewed form, in quantity just enough to hold a mixture together

- Ganache, the recipe is given below

- Fruit 3–4 cups, as per choice (might be raspberries, strawberries, blackberries and blueberries)

Ganache:

- Cacao powder ½ cup

- Maple syrup ¼ cup + 2 tbsp., you might use honey, or any other sweetener, as needed

- Coconut oil ¼ cup, melted form, you might use butter

- Vanilla extract ½ teaspoon, it is optional

Directions

Combine the walnuts and the food processor dates until the mixture is crumbling, and no big parts remain. Add cocoa powder with a pinch of salt, then mix until blended. Add 1 tbsp. Of coffee or water at a time and add it enough to keep the combination together when squeezed. Press the brownie paste in a baking parchment pan or pat into a wide ½-inch-thick ring on a rimmed baking sheet. Cool for 10–20 minutes as you're cooking the ganache.

Ganache:

In a medium dish, combine the chocolate powder, the molten coconut oil, the maple syrup and the vanilla. Stir until the mixture is smooth. (If the mixture is a little bit grainy, microwave on low flame for 10–15 sec, mix until smooth.)

Mixing Brownie Pizza and Ganache:

Take the brownie from the pan and put it on the serving tray. Layer the ganache uniformly on the pizza and finish with some fresh berries. Allows 8–10 servings, based on how big the slices are. Refrigerate the remaining in an airtight bag. Brownie's alone can keep for a week. Topped with berries, it lasts depending on berries to remains fresh, typically 2–3 days.

7.2. Basic Electric Whipped Cream

Serving: 1-2

Total time: 15 mins.

Ingredients

- Aquafaba 1 cup, it is a leftover liquid obtained from cooking chickpeas

- Agave 1/4 cup

- Stand Mixer, you might take Hand Mixer

Directions

The stand mixer would take about 5 minutes to churn together, while the hand mixer would take about 10-15 mins. The Basic Whipped Cream is completely ready to be used now, so enjoy! After using, make sure to keep it in the refrigerator.

With time passing by, the whipped cream might start to transform back to Aqaba. Stirring it again will put it back as whipped cream.

7.3. Basic Electric Walnut Butter

Serving: 2

Total time: 1 hour 15 mins.

Ingredients

- Walnuts 2 cups, soaked

- Agave 1 tablespoon, in raw form (it is optional)

- Avocado oil one teaspoon (it is also optional)

- sea salt 1/2 teaspoon

Equipment

You need a blender or food processor.

Directions

Soak two cups of the walnuts in water for 1 hour, or you can soak it all overnight. Drain the spring water and discard it. Bake the nuts in the oven for ten min at 350 ° C for producing a toasted flavor; this stage is optional. Now transfer these nuts to the blender and mix until fluffy, then put the ingredients. Offer it with fruit, or you can also use a spelled rye cracker as per your choice.

7.4. Basic Electric Donuts

Serving: 6-12

Total time: 1 hour 15 mins.

Ingredients

- Garbanzo Bean Flour 3/4 cup (also called Chickpea Flour)

- Spelt Flour 3/4 cup

- Agave 3/4 cup

- Spring Water 1/4 cup

- Basic Applesauce 1/4 cup

- Grape Seed Oil 2 tsp.

- Sea Moss Gel 1 tsp.

- Sea Salt 1/2 tsp.

- Cloves 1/4 tsp., in-ground form

Directions

Mix all the ingredients, excluding the grapeseed oil, into a wide bowl and combine until well blended. Gently spray oil on the donut pan, then preheat the oven to 350 ° F.

Place the mixture in donut pans around 3/4 from the top and bakes it for 12-14 mins. Let the donuts cool down, then, if necessary, cut out the centers depending on the pan's form. Top up with basic frosting, or you may use glaze with coconut flakes. Serve and enjoy.

7.5. Basic Electric Brazil nut Delicious Cheesecake

Serving: 6-8

Total time: 5-6 hours

Ingredients

Cheesecake Mixture:

- Brazil Nuts 2 cups

- Hemp Milk 1 1/2 cups or you may use Walnut Milk

- Agave 1/4 cup

- Dates 5-6

- Lime Juice 2 tbsp.

- Sea Moss Gel 1 tbsp.

- Sea Salt 1/4 tsp.

Crust:

- Dates 1 1/2 cups

- Coconut Flakes 1 1/2 cups

- Agave 1/4 cup

- Sea Salt 1/4 tsp.

Toppings:

- Mango, chopped

- Strawberries, chopped

- Raspberries, chopped

- Blueberries, fresh

- Blackberries, fresh

Equipment:

- Blender

- Parchment Paper

- Food Processor

- Spring-form Pan 8-inch

Directions

Put all the ingredients of the crust in the food processor, then blend them for 20 seconds.

Spread the crust into a spring-shaped pan which is lined with parchment paper.

Put the finely chopped mango around the edges of the pan and then rest in the freezer.

Apply all the components of the cheesecake mixture to the blender, then blend until smooth. Apply the mixture to the crust, wrap in foil and leave to settle for 3 or 4 hours.

Remove the outline of the pan, cover it with toppings of your choice and enjoy! Making sure you put the leftover food in the fridge!

7.6. Spelt Waffle

Serving: 4

Total time: 25 mins.

Ingredients:

- Spelt Flour 1 cup

- Sea Moss 1 tsp.

- Hemp Milk ¼ cup

- Sea Salt a pinch

- Allspice Powder ½ tsp.

Directions

To start with, whisk the oil on the waffle maker. Now preheat the waffle maker swiftly. Next, dump the dough into the maker. Lastly, cook the waffles around five to six mins over medium flame or until browned. Only serve it warm

7.7. Blueberry Cake

Serving: 6

Total time: 55 mins.

Ingredients:

- Chickpea Flour 1 cup

- Blueberries 1 cup

- Spelt Flour 2/3 cup + 1 tbsp.

- Sea Salt a pinch

- Water ¾ cup

- Grapeseed Oil 2 tbsp

- Agave Nectar 6 tbsp.

Directions

First, put all the ingredients you need to cook in a blender, then blend for three minutes until there are no more chunks in it. Next, move the paste to parchment baking pan which must be proper paper-lined and distribute it uniformly. Bake for about twenty-eight to thirty minutes or when golden browned and baked. Enjoy!

7.8. Banana Nut Muffins

Serving: 12 slices

Total time: 50 mins.

Ingredients:

- Spelt Flour 3 ½ cup
- Bananas 3, mash them
- Spring Water, as desired
- Walnuts 1 cup, sliced
- Salt a Pinch
- Date Syrup 1 tbsp.
- Perrier ¾ cup

Directions

To produce this wonderful cake, add the mashed banana and the date syrup in the bowl and mix it until well. Mix in spelled flour, then add salt and mix until combined.

Mix it again. And mix the Perrier and the walnuts. Stir it well. If the batter appears to be too dense, add a little water as required. Now add the mixture into the molds of the muffin and line them with 3/4. Lastly, bake at 350 p.m. for about eighteen to twenty minutes or till it is bake.

7.9. Blueberry Spelt Pancakes

Serving: 2

Total time: 20 mins.

Ingredients:

- Spelt Flour 2 cups

- Sea Moss ¼ tsp.

- Hemp Milk 1 cup

- Agave Syrup ½ cup

- Spring Water ½ cup

- Blueberries ½ cup

- Grapeseed Oil 2 tbsp.

Directions

For this balanced breakfast dish, add the spelled flour, the agave syrup, the sea moss and the grapeseed oil uniformly in a big mixing pot. Now, slowly pour the hemp milk into it and the water into it. Then gently press in the blueberries. After that, heat a broad pan over medium-high flame. Once the pan is hot, spray it with oil. Then, add a spoon full of the mixture and cook every side for about 3 to 5 minutes. Now finally, serve them hot.

7.10. Whipped Cream

Serving: 1

Total time: 15 mins.

Ingredients:

- Aquafaba 1 cup

- Agave Syrup ¼ cup

Directions

First, take the agave syrup and aquafaba in a small-medium size bowl and then mix them. Whisk the paste with a hand blender for about 10 to 15 minutes just until the cream becomes smooth.

7.11. Blackberry Jam

Serving: 1

Total time: 15 mins.

Ingredients:

- Blackberries ¾ cup, fresh

- Sea Moss Gel ¼ cup

- Key Lime Juice 1 tbsp.

- Agave Syrup 3 tbsp.

Directions

Begin by putting the fresh blackberries in the medium-sized bowl over medium-high flame. Stirring constantly until you have a liquid mixture. When the berries have been soft, combine them in the processor until the batter is smooth and have no chunks.

Now, put the mixture back in the pot. Then take the sea moss gel with agave syrup, stir them with lime juice and add to the mixture. Next, boil the mixture until when it gets thickens. Stir it constantly. Take the pot out of the heat and let it cool down. Serve and love yourself

7.12. Dates Ball

Serving: makes 24 balls

Total time: 50 mins.

Ingredients:

- Walnuts ½ cup

- Sea Salt ½ tsp.

- Dates 1 cup, little bit pitted

- Agave Syrup ¼ cup

- Coconut Meat 1 cup

- Sesame Seeds ½ cup

Directions

Start by putting all the ingredients, excluding sesame seeds, in the processor and then blend them five times for about 20 seconds. Then switch the paste to a wide dish. Now, keep the balls out from the dish. Then dunk these balls in the sesame coats and then cover them deeply. Serve and love yourself.

7.13. Sweetened Chickpeas

Serving: 1

Total time: 50 mins.

Ingredients:

- Garbanzo Beans 15 oz., rinsed, drained & dry

- Agave Syrup 2 tbsp.

- Sea Salt ½ tsp.

- Olive Oil 1 tbsp.

Directions

Start with preheating the oven to 350 ft. Then add with the garbanzo beans, the sea salt, and the olive oil and agave syrup in a large mixing pan. Then mix well. Now move the paste into a baking tray lined with parchment paper, then distribute it thinly in a single sheet. Finally, bake for about 45 minutes, or when become crispy

7.14. Raisin Cookies

Servings: 2

Total Time: 45 Minutes

Ingredients:

- Applesauce 2/3 cup
- Raisins 1 cup
- Spelt Flour 1 ½ cup
- Pure Sea Salt ½ tsp.
- rolled Spelt flakes, 1 ½ cup
- Grapeseed Oil 1/3 cup
- Spring Water 2 tbsp.
- Dates pitted 1 ½ cup
- Agave 1/3 cup

Direction

To make these tasty cookies, all you need is to mix the spelled first. Add sea salt with dates into a food processor. Next, move the wheat mixture into a large bowl and then add the flour mixture. Add the spelled flakes. After that, blend all the remaining items and add them to the mixture. Have a good mix till you get a dough. Now, create the balls of dough and place them on a parchment baker's sheet. Make the balls flatten with a fork. Finally, bake them at 350 F about 20 minutes.

7.15. Banana Walnut Ice Cream

Servings: 4

Total Time: 15 Minutes

Ingredients:

- Strawberries 1 cup
- chopped Avocado ½ of 1,

- Walnut Milk ¼ cup

- quartered Baby Bananas, 5

- Agave Syrup 1 tbsp.

Directions:

Start by adding all the ingredients into a high-speed blender you to make ice cream for 2 minutes. Add more walnut milk in case it is too thick. Then move the mixture to a broad freezer-safe tub. Then freeze it for 4 hours till it's set.

7.16. Walnut Date Nog

Servings: 2

Total Time: 10 Minutes

Ingredients:

- chopped Walnuts, ¼ cup

- Sea Salt ½ tsp.

- soaked Dates 4

- grounded Clove 1

- Hemp Seeds 4 tbsp.

- Dash of Anise

- Agave Syrup 2 tbsp.

- Spring Water 18 oz.

Directions:

Start by putting all the ingredients required to create the nog, except the clove and anise, inside a high-speed blender. Blend for about three minutes or till the mixture is smooth. Next, move the mixture into a medium-sized saucepan and heat. Serve with a slice of clove or anise. Enjoy it.

7.17. Mango Cheesecake

Servings: 8

Total Time: 4 Hour 30 Minutes

Ingredients:

- Walnut Milk 1 ½ cup
- Brazil Nuts 2 cups
- Pure Sea Salt ¼ tsp.
- Dates 6
- Lime Juice 2 tbsp.
- Sea Moss 1 tbsp.
- Agave Syrup ¼ cup

For crust:

- Agave Syrup 1/4 cup
- Sea Salt ¼ tsp.
- quartered Dates 1 ½ cup,
- Coconut Flakes 1 ½ cup

Directions:

First, put all the ingredients necessary to make the dough into a food processor, then process for 30 -45 minutes. Place the mixture onto the parchment paper-lined baking dish. Now distribute the mixture uniformly over the sheet. Then place mango slices over the crust and put it inside the freezer for 8-10 minutes. Meanwhile, put filling ingredients into a high-speed blender. Blend until the mixture is smooth. Next, dump the mixture all over the frozen surface and let it stay in the refrigerator for 3-4 hours. Finally, before serving, garnish with some more slices of mango and strawberries

7.18. Strawberry Sorbet

Servings: 4

Total Time: 4 hours 10 minutes

Ingredients:

- Date Sugar ½ cup
- Strawberries 2 cups
- Spring Water 2 cups
- Spelt Flour 1 ½ tsp.

Directions:

Begin by combing date sugar, spelled flour, and spring water in a medium-sized pot. Next, heat the mixture over low heat and cook for 8 to 10 minutes or till thickened. After that, take off the pot from the heat and allow it to cool. Once cooled, puree the strawberries in a blender. Now, mix the strawberry puree to the flour mixture and give everything a good stir. Then, pour the mixture into a container and keep it in the freezer. Cut the frozen sorbet to pieces and place it in the blender or food processor. Blend until smooth and return the container to the refrigerator for a minimum of 4 hours.

Finally, serve the chilled strawberry sorbet.

7.19. Strawberry Ice Cream

Servings: 3 to 4

Total Time: 6 hours 10 Minutes

Ingredients:

- Hemp Milk ¼ cup
- frozen strawberries, 1 cup
- Agave Syrup 1 tbsp.
- frozen Baby Bananas, 5

- ripe Avocado, ½ of 1

Directions:

Place all ingredients necessary to make this ice cream into a high-speed blender. Mix them for 2-3 minutes or till the mixture is smooth. Check for sugar and, if appropriate, insert more agave syrup. Finally, move to the freezer-friendly jar and freeze for 4-6 hours

Chapter 8: Dr. Sebi's shakes

8.1. Sherbet Mango Coconut

Serving: 4

Total Time: 15 minutes

Ingredients:

- Sweet mangoes 2

- Agave Nectar¼ cup

- Raw Coconut Milk, ½ cup

Directions:

You must first ice the mangoes to produce this tasty sherbet. Freeze for eight hours in the fridge. When frozen, mix 2 - 3 minutes in a high-speed mixer. Or until it's smooth. Drop the milk from the cocoa agave nectar and combine until melted again. You will get a smooth sherbet Serve right away.

8.2. Mashed Squash

Serving:6

Total Time: 10 minutes

Ingredients:

- Blue Agave (organic) ¼ cup

- Squash, 2 cut into chunks

- Pure Sea Salt 1/8 tsp.

- Date Sugar ¼ cup

- Hemp Milk ¼ cup

Directions:

To start, put the squash pieces in a pot and add water from the spring. Over low heat, give the mixture a boil and simmer for 20 mins. It's becoming tender. Drain the water until tender and take it out. Add a Spoon of sugar, some sea salt, any spice of choice but approved, and hemp milk.

8.3. Quinoa Pear Smoothie

Serving: 1

Total Time: 10minute

Ingredients:

- pitted Avocado, ¼ of 1
- Spring Water1 cup
- cooked Quinoa, ¼ cup
- Spring Water 1 cup
- Blueberries 1 oz.
- Pear1

Directions:

To produce this smoothie, add ingredients in a high-speed mixer, blend for 3 mins. Or until it is fluffy and smooth. Pour into a glass bottle and enjoy it.

8.4. Papaya Smoothie

Serving: 1

Total Time: 10 minutes

Ingredients:

- Coconut Milk ½ cup
- Papaya 1 cup
- Lime Juice 1 tsp.
- Strawberries 4
- Frozen Pineapple, ½ cup

- Ginger ¼-inch

Directions:

Place all the requisite ingredients for making papaya smoothie start blending for 2 minutes in a high-speed mixer. Pour into a serving glass when it's smooth and luscious.

8.5. Banana Ginger Smoothie

Serving:1

Total Time: 10 minutes

Ingredients:

- Frozen Banana 1,

- Agave Syrup 1 tbsp.

- Hemp Milk 2 cups

- chopped Strawberries ½ cup,

- Kale 1

- The ginge1-inch piece, finely minced

Directions:

Begin by combining all ingredients in a high-speed mixer, blend or 5 Minutes or till smooth without any chunks. Serve and drink it.

8.6. Orange Berry Smoothie

Serving: 1

Total Time: 10 minutes

Ingredients:

- Burro Banana1medium size

- Berries 1 cup

- Seville Orange 1

- Ripe Avocado, ¼ of 1

- Fresh Lettuce, 2 cups

- Spring Water, as required

- Hemp Seeds 1 tbsp.

Directions:

To create this tasty smoothie, combine all ingredients. Combine all ingredients for 2 to 3 minutes in a high-speed mixer till you get a rich and delicious smoothie.

8.7. Watermelon and Cucumber Smoothie

Serving: 1

Total Time: 10

Ingredients:

- Cucumber1

- cubed Watermelon, 1cup

- Key Lime1

Directions:

Place the watermelon, cucumber and key lime first at a really fast pace. Use for 1-2 minutes blender, or until a smooth mixture is reached. Now step into a bottle to indulge.

8.8. Pear Smoothie

Serving: 1

Total Time: 10 minutes

Ingredients:

- cooked Quinoa, ¼ cup

- chopped 1 Pear,

- Blueberries1 oz.

- pitted Avocado ¼ of 1,

- Water1 cup

Directions:

To create this tasty smoothie, combine all ingredients. Combine all ingredients for 2 to 3 minutes in a high-speed mixer till you get a rich and delicious smoothie.

8.9. Detox Green Smoothie

Serving: 1

Total Time: 10 minutes

Ingredients:

- Greens Amaranth 2 cups

- Spring Water 2 cups

- Key Lime 1

- cored Apples, 2

- cubed Avocado, ¼ of 1

Directions:

- Put the greens, and avocado, with apple and key lime, high-speed blender adds appropriate amount of water. Blend the mixture for 1 to 1 ½ minutes, just before you get a rich and well-blended mixture. Serve and have fun.

8.10. Tomato Cucumber Smoothie

Serving: 1

Total Time: 10 minutes

Ingredients:

- Cucumber 1

- Agave Syrup3 tbsp.

- Plum Tomato 1

- Water 2 cups

Directions:

To create this tasty smoothie, combine all ingredients. Combine all ingredients for 2 to 3 minutes in a high-speed mixer till you get a rich and delicious smoothie.

8.11. Peach Berry Smoothie

Serving: 1

Total Time: 10 minutes

Ingredients:

- Sea Moss1 tbsp.

- Coconut Milk 1 cup

- Strawberries ½ cup

- Hemp Seeds 1 tbsp.

- quartered½ Peaches, cup

- Agave Syrup1 tbsp.

- Blueberries ½ cup

Directions:

Put bananas and agave syrup in a blender, add sea moss, hemp seed and coconut Milk, with blueberries and peaches in a high-speed blender. Blend the mixture for 1 minute or till you have a nice and luxurious smoothie. Transfer to the serving glass, drink instantly. Enjoy it!

8.12. Watermelon Smoothie

Serving: 1

Total Time: 10 minutes

Ingredients:

- Coconut Water 1 cup
- Pieces of Watermelon 1 cup
- Date Syrup 1 tbsp.
- Strawberries 1 cup

Directions:

Start by blending the watermelon and strawberries, then add coconut water and, finally, the dates. Blend in a high-speed blender for almost 1-2 minutes or till you get a smooth and rich mixture. Transfer to a glass. Enjoy!

8.13. Berry Walnut Smoothie

Serving: 2

Total Time: 10

Ingredients:

- Raw Walnuts 1 cup, Soaked at least 8 hours
- Coconut Milk ½ cup
- Figs 2, soaked for about 8 hours
- Key Lime Juice 1 tbsp

- Strawberries ¼ cup

- Agave Syrup 1 tsp.

Directions:

Start by placing all the ingredients into a blender to create this perfect smoothie. Mix everything for 3 mins. Or until smooth. Move to the serving glass with the topping of nuts authorized by Dr. Sebi.

8.14. Apple Smoothie

Serving: 2

Total Time: 25

Ingredients:

- Sea Moss1 tbsp.

- Ice 2 cups

- fresh Apple Juice, 2 cups

- Ginger1 tbsp.

- Clove Powder A Dash

Directions:

Place all ingredients as needed to create this perfect smoothie. Start blending for making a smoothie in a high-speed blender. Blend for 1 ½ minutes or till you have a creamy smoothie. Now, stir with the ice and blend for another minute. In the end, move to a serving glass.

8.15. Cucumber Coconut Smoothie

Serving: 1

Total Time: 10 minutes

Ingredients:

- Cucumbers 2

- Agave Nectar 1 tsp.

- Young Coconut 1

- Ginger 1-inch

Directions:

To create this tasty smoothie, combine all ingredients. Combine all ingredients for 2 to 3 minutes in a high-speed mixer till you get a rich and delicious smoothie.

8.16. Green Monster Smoothie

Serving: 1

Total Time: 10 minutes

Ingredients:

- Avocado, ½ of 1

- Diced Mango ½ of 1

- Dates pitted 2-3

- Sour soup Pulp 1 tbsp.

- Rainbow Kale 1 Bunch, without leaves

- Coconut Water ½ cup

Directions:

Create this tasty smoothie, combine all ingredients. Blend all ingredients for 2 to 3 minutes in a high-speed mixer. Serve with ice on the top glass.

8.17. Strawberry Banana Smoothie

Serving: 2

Total Time: 10 minutes

Ingredients:

- Hemp Milk 2 cups

- 4 Banana

- Strawberry 8 oz.

- Dates ¾ cup

- Agave1 tbsp.

Directions:

You need to start by putting the strawberries in a blender to create this tasty smoothie. Mix the strawberries and other ingredients for a minute or two in a blender, or before they are slightly broken down. Then add banana and hemp milk. After that, put agave. Blend for 2-3 minutes or till well mixed. Enjoy it!

Chapter 9: Dr. Sebi's Sauces

9.1. Tomato Pizza Sauce

Serving: 2

Total Time: 5 minutes

Ingredients:

- Roma Tomatoes 5
- chopped Onion 2 tbs
- Sea Salt 1 tsp.
- Onion Powder 1 tsp.
- Oregano1 tsp.
- Agave 2 tbsp.
- Grapeseed Oil 2 tbsp.
- Basil a pinch

Directions:

Make x-shaped small cuts on ends of five plum tomatoes to peel the skin and put them into boiling water for 1 min. Shake tomatoes in ice-cold water for up to 30 seconds so that the skin can be quickly peeled. Mix tomatoes with other ingredients into the food processor or a blender for 30 sec. or until smooth.

9.2. Avocado Pizza Sauce

Serving: 2

Total Time: 7 minutes

Ingredients:

- Onion Chopped 2 tbsp.
- Onion Powder 1/2 tsp.

- Sea Salt 1/2 tsp.

- Oregano 1/2 tsp.

- Basil a pinch

Directions:

Break down the avocado from the middle, remove the seed, and clean the interior of your food processor. Add remaining of the ingredients into a food processor, blend for 3 min. or till smooth.

9.3. Avocado Sauce with Zoodle

Serving: 2

Total Time: 20 minutes

Ingredients:

- Zucchinis 2 large

- Basil 2 cups

- Water 1/2 cup

- Walnuts 1/2 cup

- Key lime juice 4 tbsp

- Avocados 2

- Cherry tomatoes sliced24

- Sea salt as per your taste

Directions:

Use a peeler or Spiralizer to produce zucchini noodles. Mix all ingredients (except cherry tomatoes) into the blender until smooth. Use a mixing dish, add pasta, after that add cherry tomatoes and finally the avocado sauce.

9.4. Alkaline Electric Tzatziki & Falafel Sauce

Serving: 2-4

Total Time: 40 minutes

Ingredients:

For Falafel

- garbanzo beans cooked 2 cups
- garbanzo bean flour 1/2 cup
- chopped onions cup 1/2
- aquafaba 1/3 cup (remaining water collected from cooked chickpeas)
- chopped green onions, 1/4 cup
- Alkaline "Garlic" Sauce 2 tbsp.
- Lime juice 1 tbsp.
- Tahini 1 tbsp.
- oregano 1 tsp
- Basil 1 tsp.
- Onion powder 1 tsp.
- Sea salt 1/2 tsp.
- Cayenne 1/2 tsp.
- grapeseed oil
- food processor

Tzatziki Sauce

- Brazil nuts cup 1/2, (Soak nuts 6-8 hours into spring water, then for 1-2 hours into hot water)
- Aquafaba 1/3 cup
- chopped cucumber, 1/4 cup

- Springwater 2 tbsp.

- Lime juice 1 tbsp.

- Alkaline "Garlic" Sauce 1 tbsp.

- Fresh dill 1 tsp.

- sea salt a pinch

Directions:

Add all of the falafel ingredients into the food processor (except oil) and blend them until well-blended. The mixture is supposed to be cooked until you can turn the mixture into a ball. Add more flour in case the mixture is too wet. Heat up to 1 tablespoon of oil (Grapeseed) in a skillet over medium heat. Cook the falafel balls from each side for about 4-5 minutes, flipping tongs. Bake the falafel at 400 ° F for around 5 to 10 minutes.

Add all the tzatziki sauce components, then add 1 tbsp of the water into the blender, blend for about 1 minute. If required, add more water. You may eat falafel with Alkaline-Electric-Hummus; you may also make falafel salad or make a gyro with the Alkaline-Electric-Flatbread, hummus, or tzatziki sauce and a variety of vegetables.

9.6. Alkaline Electric Hot Sauce

Serving:

Total Time:

Ingredients:

- Habaneros 3*

- Springwater 1/3 cup

- Red Pepper 1/4 cup

- Diced Onions, 1/4 cup

- Sea Salt 1/2 tsp

- Onion Powder 1 tbsp.

- Lime Juice 2 tbsp

- Grape Seed Oil 1 tbsp.

Directions:

*Don't forget to cook the habaneros whole. While cooking, makes sure to maintain proper ventilation because these peppers are powerful. Add the grape-seed oil into the skillet over medium heat. Add garlic, tomatoes, onions and habaneros to the skillet and Sautee them for 3-4 minutes. Remove the habanero roots, then add vegetables with all the other ingredients into the blender. Mix until the sauce becomes creamy, and strain the seeds. Enjoy hot sauce.

9.7. Applesauce

Serving: 2

Total Time: 5 minutes

Ingredients:

- Sea Moss Gel 1 tsp.

- chopped Apples, 3cups

- Pure Sea Salt 1/8 tsp.

- Agave Syrup 3 tbsp.

- Cloves 1/8 tsp.

- Lime Juice 1 tsp.

- Spring Water, as required

Directions:

To create this tasty sauce, combine all ingredients in a high-speed blender. Cook on medium heat for about 2 minutes. Blend another time all ingredients for 2 to 3 minutes in a high-speed mixer till you get a rich and delicious sauce.

9.8. Avocado Yoghurt Sauce

Serving: 2

Total Time: 10 minutes

Ingredients:

- Agave Syrup 1/3 cup

- Ripe Avocado 1,

- Spring Water ¾ cup

- Juice of 2 Limes

- Berries 1 cup

Directions:

Begin with agave sipping, berries, spring water, and lime juice. Use a high-speed mixer with avocado in it. Blend it for 1-2 minutes, till no chunks or until smooth. Serve when cooled.

9.9. Mango salsa

Serving: 3

Total Time: 10 minutes

Ingredients:

- Plum Tomatoes, 6

- Cayenne Pepper ½ tsp.

- Tomatillo 1

- Sea Salt1 tsp

- chopped Red Onion ½ cup,

- Onion Powder 1 tsp

- Green Bell Pepper ¼ cup

- Cilantro ½ cup

- ½ cup Mango,

- Juice of a half Lemon

Directions:

Start by mixing all required ingredients except salsa into the food processor with pineapple. Treat them for 10-15 seconds; add the mango then. Scrap the sides, mix again for 20 seconds.

Take a cup and enjoy.

9.10. Salsa Verde

Serving: 2

Total Time: 10

Ingredients:

- Cilantro ¼ cup

- Onion Powder 1 tsp.

- Tomatillo, 1 lb. must be washed and skin removed.

- Pure Sea Salt 1 tsp.

- diced Onion ½ cup,

- Oregano 1 tsp.

Directions:

Start by putting the onions along with other ingredients to create this tasty dip. On Medium heat except for cilantro in a pan and fill it with water. Cook this mixture for 20 minutes, then stir from time to time. Then add the juice using a strainer. Next, transfer this whole mixture into a high-speed blender. Blend the mixture for about half a minute.

9.11. BBQ Sauce

Serving: 1

Total Time: 45 minutes

Ingredients:

- Cloves 1/8 tsp.

- Plum Tomatoes, 6

- Pure Sea Salt 2 tsp.

- chopped Onion, ¼ cup

- Onion Powder 2 tsp.

- Cayenne¼ tsp.

- Date Sugar ¼ cup

- Agave Syrup 2 tbsp.

Directions:

First, put all the ingredients required to make this sauce in a Mixer for high-speed. Mix them for 1-2 minutes or till a smooth paste is produced. Now pass the mixture into the tiny cup and drain date sugar from it. Cook on medium heat and mix regularly. Next, the heat should be low and allow the mixture to simmer for 15 minutes covered with a lid. Remember to stir frequently. Then mix in a blender until you get a smooth mixture using an immersion blender. Transfer the sauce again to the casserole and cook for another 10 minutes more. Let it cool down and then store.

9.12. Tomato Sauce

Serving: 6

Total Time: 45 minutes

Ingredients:

- Basil 3 tsp.

- Cayenne Pepper 1/8 tsp.

- Halved Roma Tomatoes, 18.

- Basil 3 tsp.

- halved Sweet Onion, ½ of 1

- Onion Powder 2 tsp.

- halved Red Onion, ½ of 1

- halved Bell Pepper, diced ½ of 1

- Agave Syrup 1 tbsp.

- Oregano 2 tsp.

- Pure Sea Salt 3 tsp.

- Grape-seed Oil 1/8 cup

Directions:

Get ready to preheat your oven to 400 ° F. Then put the vegetables in a large pot. To this end, add a teaspoon of grapevine oil and 100% pure sea salt, then add Basil and toss well.

Put the coated vegetables into a greased baking dish. Then roast the vegetables for about 25 to 30 minutes. Now turn the sheet in the middle. After roasting, bring the vegetables into a blender and blend them. For one minute or till a smooth paste is obtained. Finally, move the mixture into a medium-sized saucepan over medium heat. Then simmer for another twenty minutes. Serve and enjoy.

9.13 Hot Sauce

Serving: 1

Total Time: 35 minutes

Ingredients:

- Sea Moss Powder 1 tbsp.

- Spring Water 1 ½ cups

- Onion Powder 2 tbsp.

- Key Lime Juice ½ cup

- Cayenne Pepper 2 tbsp.

- Plum Tomatoes 9

- Pure Sea Salt ½ tsp.

Directions:

Start with all ingredients to create the hot sauce. Mix and blend it in a high-speed blender for 3 minutes or before you obtain a smooth paste. Then heat this mixture over medium heat. Cook the mixture around 10-15 minutes, then let it cool. Store in a glass jar. Snacks and bread based on Doctor Sebi products.

9.14. Spelt Bread

Serving: 4

Total Time: 1 hour & 10 minutes

Ingredients:

- Pure Sea Salt 2 tsp.

- Spelt Flour 4 ½ cup

- Agave Syrup ¼ cup

- Sesame Seeds 1 tsp.

- Grape Seed Oil 2 tsp.

- Spring Water 2 cups

Directions:

First, put the spelt-flour with sea salt into a food processor for 10-20 seconds. Add agave syrup and blend properly. Then add a spoon of oil and some water to get dough, then steadily mix. Process this dough for another five minutes. Holding the dough in the aggregated and distorted loaf. Preheat an oven to 350 F. Allow it to stay for 1 hour. Finally, bake until golden brown for 50- 60 minutes.

9.15. Chickpeas Cornbread

Serving: 14

Total Time: 25 minutes

Ingredients:

- Chickpea Flour 2 cup
- Brazil Nut Milk 1 cup
- Applesauce 1 cup
- Water, as required
- Grapeseed Oil ½ cup
- Pepper 1 tbsp.

Directions:

Start combining in large mixing bowl all necessary ingredients for making the cornbread smooth. It should be moderately consistent. If the batter is too thickened, you may also use water to dilute it. Place the grapefruit oil in the pot and add the butter to it.

Disseminate it uniformly. Bake for 28-30 minutes or till toothpick comes out clean if inserted in the batter. Cut into squares until cooled. After it gets cool, slice into squares.

9.16. Zucchini Bread

Serving: 2

Total Time: 45 minutes

Ingredients:

- Oil 2 tbsp.
- Zucchini Puree 1 cup
- Spelt Flour 1 cup
- Pinch of Salt
- Perrier 1 tbsp.

Directions:

Start mixing the puree with the rice, milk, salt and the Perrier spelt. Until all comes together into a large mixing bowl, pour some more water to obtain a dense and smooth dough. Now stretched the dough on a grated paper baker sheet. Bake the dough at 350 F for 33 mins. Or until cooked.

9.17. Alkaline Electric Breadsticks

Serving: 2

Total Time: 45 minutes

Ingredients:

- Spelt Flour 2 cups

- spring Water3/4 cup

- Alkaline "Garlic" Sauce* 1/2 cup

- Agave 2 tsp.

- Onion Powder 1 tbsp.

- Sea Salt half of 1 tsp.

- Oregano 1 tsp.

- Basil 1 tsp.

- Grounded Brazil Nuts 1/4 cup (Optional)

- Garlic sauce, 1/4 cup in 2 cups separately.

Directions:

Add the flour to the mixer and blend for 30 seconds. Put agave into the mixer, knead the pasta for 5 minutes, and then add 1/4 cup of alkaline garlic sauce with water. Wrap in plastic lightly flour dough ball, let the dough stay for 30 minutes. Remove a small portion of the dough using a dough cutter, roll it back and forth with soft hands. Put together dough ends, twist until long enough, and then position it on a bakery pan. Brush the 1/4 cup of alkaline 'garlic' sauce gently on the breadsticks and bake for 15 min, at 350 ° F.

Grind with coffee grinder the Brazil nuts until it is finely ground. Once brushed, add the remaining sauce into the breadsticks, now top with ground Brazil nozzles and bake for 3 minutes. Enjoy your fresh Electric Alkaline Breadstick.

Chapter 10: Training strategy

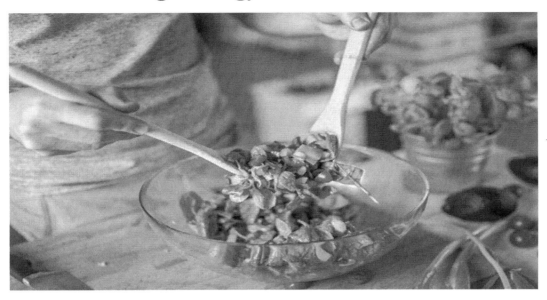

Getting Ready for Dr. Sebi Diet.

Since first beginning following Sebi's and telling friends and family regarding his plans, most of them seem to have reservations that one might not adjust to such a diet and lifestyle. But here for the 6th year, and its always going high.

Like other people, everybody I spoke to looked at things the wrong way – concentrating on the drawbacks of the food rather than possibilities. I guess the biggest explanation for this is that, for those living on fast food and pre-packaged garbage, much of the food in Sebi's list may sound a little foreign because there's a lot of stuff out there by using which you can create hearty meals.

Now, it depends on where you are with your overall dietary behaviors at the moment. Following a Sebian way to eat may involve some serious adjustments. If you're still vegan, it'll be mainly smooth sailing. However, if you like to eat a lot of meat and fast food (like me), transitioning to this diet would take a lot of work on your end.

My tips on people trying to follow a Sebi diet are simple. Below, I'm going to go through the key stuff I wish anyone had taught me when I first began doing this years ago. Anyways if you're still not sure what this diet means to take a peek at my webpage. I'm providing a rundown, along with some advantages.

Be armed physically and psychologically to fully adjust to Serbian's eating style. You may have to begin by making certain adjustments to your overall lifestyle. You're likely to discover that this allows people to be in the correct state of mind and mental condition.

Eating is part of life, and the kinds of foods or drugs we eat daily shape solid behaviors that will last for a lifetime if we left them unchecked.

These patterns may be incredibly difficult to overcome or alter. The power of the culture and people nearest to us may also be a hindrance.

That's why, before you rush into this diet style, you can take more time dreaming about improving your food don't pledge something then just struggle because of lack of planning, family problems, or something, then break something pledge.

Start consuming some of the water is important to cleanse your bodies, sustain balanced brain or body functions, with a variety of other benefits.

A variety of Sebi products, like his Bromide-Plus-Powder, include herbs, including Bladderwrack, containing laxative properties and encourage urination to eliminate contaminants. Hence, you need to consume enough water to refill it and always keep you hydrated.

It recommends consuming up to 1 gallon of fresh spring water a day. Springwater is preferred since it is usually alkaline instead of tap water, rich in chlorine and other toxins.

Begin reading the ingredients labels. It's not going to be convenient for certain people to give-up those sweets or soft beverages. Hence, a perfect way to get started is to scan the food product labels. It's a great idea and an utter requirement to be mindful of what you're consuming and drinking. At first, if you don't eat based on the food chart, this knowledge may allow you to improve your behaviors as you advance.

Snacking in the best way. Snacking may be a compulsive activity, but it doesn't suggest it has to be a poor one. Most people enjoy snacks many times, but instead of finding a bag full of chips or a big chocolate bar, why not consider making your snacks mix of walnuts and raisins along with other dried fruits.

Add more natural grains to the current diet. Start incorporating more whole foods into your current diet regularly. Don't think so much if it's not vegan food. At this point, it's more crucial that you take any sort of steps to improve what you're consuming to avoid depending on unhealthy food or quick food. There could be anything of your choice, from berries to a new fish fillet. The key goal here is to eat more natural foods instead of processed foods made of chemicals. Avoiding these ingredients can benefit you later on in your journey since all of these products are addictive. Refined sugar is highly addictive and induces food cravings.

When you pass the line from packaged eating to cooking every day, the road to health rehabilitation and control gets even smoother. You can soon see the countless possibilities available and learn how you can take your beloved recipes and re-make them like accepted recipes to experience the same meals you've always had.

Begin eating Irish moss: Get associated with Irish sea-moss try producing a gel. This is one of your diet pillars because it's healthy and it's tasteless, so you can apply it to any of your favorite meals without really knowing it's there.

Introduce authorized foods from Dr. Sebi. When you're finished, print out the food list and select a couple of foods you know about, replacing whatever you can with products on in list from your current diet.

Empower yourself with some recipes authorized by Sebi.

I've already put together a compilation of easy to prepare Sebi's approved recipes. Now I recommend you take a couple of them and start replacing some of the traditional meals every week.

Conclusion

Dr. Sebi ties the connections between physical and mental disorders and nutrition. A skeletal human, anyone lacking in vitamins and nutrients, has a brain that breaks down, resulting in irrational thought and, eventually, dangerous behavior. If the body gets everything it wants, it's calm. Healing the intestines by eliminating contaminants is related to healing the brain. A toxin is removed from an alkaline diet devoid of acid-based foods. Happiness is affected if the organism is acidic. When the body is extremely acidic, instability, madness, discontent, and aggression occur.

Follow the pattern of life: design. We get phosphates, carbonates, iodides, and bromide from nature. They are regarded as food by biochemistry. If we consume the right stuff, we don't require nutritionists. Elephants, lions and all species have no nutritionists. Consequently, foods dependent on starch are clinically referred to as carbonic acid. It causes a reaction that releases a sculpture that robs the body of oxygen. We have to consume electrical food to get an electrical body. Electrical food enables absorption and assimilation. Healing includes any part of man. Healing promotes healing because there will be no healing until there is well-being in the body. This Book concludes here with the message that life is beautiful don't waste it by consuming food which is not good for your well-being. Start following Dr. Sebi diet to spend a great and healthy life.

Printed in Great Britain
by Amazon

57300509R00070